EVERY WOMAN'S GUIDE TO FOOT PAIN RELIEF

EVERY WOMAN'S GUIDE TO FOOT PAIN RELIEF

The New Science of Healthy Feet

KATY BOWMAN, MS

BenBella Books, Inc.
Dallas, Texas

BenBella

BenBella Books, Inc.
10300 N. Central Expressway
Suite #400
Dallas, TX 75231
benbellabooks.com
Send feedback to feedback@benbellabooks.com

Printed in the United States of America
10 9 8 7 6 5 4 3 2 1

Library of Congress Cataloging-in-Publication Data is available for this title.
ISBN 978-1-936661-07-7

Editing by Erin Kelley
Copyediting by Lisa Miller
Proofreading by Michael Fedison and Nora Nussbaum
Cover design by Kit Sweeney
Text design and composition by Silver Feather Design
Printed by Berryville Graphics

Distributed by Perseus Distribution • perseusdistribution.com
To place orders through Perseus Distribution:
Tel: 800-343-4499
Fax: 800-351-5073
E-mail: orderentry@perseusbooks.com

Significant discounts for bulk sales are available. Please contact Glenn Yeffeth at glenn@benbellabooks.com or (214) 750-3628.

DEDICATION

For Theresa, who leaves two sets of
aligned foot prints wherever she goes.

TABLE OF CONTENTS

CHAPTER 1

How much do you know about your own anatomy? Did you know that you should be able to lift each toe by itself? Can you? If not, the basics of foot motion will be a fun ride!

CHAPTER 2

Any ballerinas out there walking around with their feet turned out? Why do our gait patterns differ so greatly from person to person, but tend to be the same within a family? (Hint: it's not genetic!)

CHAPTER 3

Sometimes foot pain is created much higher in your body than you realize. The way you stand can load tissue in the wrong place, causing it to wear out before its time. Do you wear your hips out in front of you? That's a good place to start looking for likely culprits!

CHAPTER 4

Even though bunions tend to run in a family, their appearance in your family tree has a lot more to do with the way you learned to move your body and the footwear you are choosing to wear, as opposed to flaws in your tissue. Find a solution here!

CHAPTER 5

Your Shoes...a Map

The parts of a shoe go beyond the latest style. By learning to identify four main characteristics, you can make smart choices when it comes to improving your outfit—and your foot health.

CHAPTER 6

Shoe Science

What is it about a shoe, really, that limits foot health? Turns out that the four main parts of a shoe each have particular qualities that can increase the development of common ailments like hammertoes, plantar fasciitis, bunions...just to name a few!

CHAPTER 7

Women...Undermining Women's Health

Is the high heel really that bad? Really? What about the research? If a shoe was implicated in ailments of the foot, knee, or spine, wouldn't it be on the front of every newspaper? Well, the research is showing something, and frankly, no one is talking!

CHAPTER 8

The Foot Gym

Everyone knows they are supposed to exercise, but few of us know what to do with the muscles in the foot...and there are a lot of them down there. This chapter offers a simple, easy-to-follow program that will help you restore function to the underused muscles in the feet, as well as increase circulation to the tight, overstressed tissue of the lower leg.

CHAPTER 9

Taking the Next (First) Step

Do healthy feet require a complete closet makeover? Am I going to be banned from cute shoes forever? How do I fit more exercise into my busy day when I can barely handle what is currently on my plate? Find those answers here.

CHAPTER 10

Guidelines, Recommendations, and
What if I don't have foot pain, but want to prevent it? What if I want to optimize foot development in my friends and family? Does footwear matter during pregnancy, childhood, and my later years? Included here are guidelines on footwear for various ages and stages in life. Come find out what is best for your (or your family's) feet!

FOREWORD

As a medical specialist of the foot and ankle, I have encountered complaints from patients suffering with a variety of problems, including corns, hammertoes, bunions, and heel pain. Any podiatrist would tell you that treatments for these conditions include orthotics, injections, padding, medications, and/or changes in shoes.

Patients have also seen me seeking a second opinion after they have been recommended a surgical procedure. The explanation usually given to the patient is that her musculoskeletal problem has become a fixed structural deformity that cannot be corrected.

In spite of the many advances in surgical treatment, we must be aware that these are biomechanical problems, and as such are inherently more dynamic than they may first appear. Realize that the majority of these problems are not congenital, and we have acquired them from a lack of knowledge regarding movement, bad habits, and many times, poor shoe selection.

In this primer on healthy foot mechanics, Katy Bowman amuses as she informs you about the many things you can do to keep your feet feeling great. She offers simple solutions that you can take advantage of and practice on your own. I have seen positive results among my patients who perform these exercises.

Ms. Bowman's approach to clinical biomechanics is novel, and it is revolutionary. Her insight into the complex area that is the foot is literally the foundation for total body wellness.

At a time of so much uncertainty regarding the future of health care, and the increasing prevalence of diseases like diabetes and obesity, you can take control of your own health by educating yourself about how your body works.

Every Woman's Guide to Foot Pain Relief is a testament to the effectiveness of specific exercise protocol to correct lower-leg ailments that are mechanical in nature. Empower yourself with this handbook; some relief may be immediate, and lasting relief may require diligence.

If Ms. Bowman is part of a revolution in how we approach our health, the new paradigm will support only those interested in taking full responsibility for their own health. As this book demonstrates, wellness is out there for those who are willing to work for it.

Dr. Theresa Perales

Podiatrist

Ventura, California

INTRODUCTION

There are many milestones along the path to well-maintained feet, and an increasingly common detour is the path to the doctor's office, pharmacy, or even the operating room to fix an ailment from the ankle down. Far from being neatly confined to your shoes, foot problems actually speak volumes about the future status of your knees and hips, ability to walk for exercise, and ultimately the ability to live your golden years as a mobile and independent person. The foot is involved in virtually every non-sitting activity we do. If we want to stay upright and active—and feel great at the same time—we need to know more about our feet.

Often people will tell me, "I am too old to make any significant improvements in my health," or, "My feet have been like this for so long, they will never change!" Both of these statements are untrue! The state of your feet right now is simply the reflection of everything you have done up until this moment. Human tissues are dynamic and adapt to the forces that are placed upon them. When these forces change, the tissues change to reflect the different habit. This is true whether it's a good habit or a bad one!

This book is about how you can fix your own feet. Although human body issues often seem complex—especially to those people with little or no anatomical, physiological, or therapeutic training—solutions can be much simpler than they appear. Though not on purpose, this "healing is complex" attitude is frequently reinforced by the entire health care system. As pharmaceutical and technological sciences advance, it makes sense that these advanced treatments would be the first used. After all, the more advanced the treatment, the better it is, right?

In actuality, most ailments do not require expensive treatments, complicated products, or even pharmaceutical intervention. Most musculoskeletal issues—that is, ailments of the bones, ligaments, tendons, and muscles—are usually created by one very simple, easily evaluated habit: *how you move.*

The relationship between *how you move* and *how your body feels* becomes more and more clear the better one understands *how things work in the body.* Inconveniently, the human body wasn't created with an easy-to-use manual for quick troubleshooting when a problem arises. But all hope is not lost. By working backward, any person with the right training in physics and geometry can figure out which joint positions create the most degeneration, which footwear choices can increase pressure on which tissues, and which patterns of gait, or walking, can reduce muscle strength and nerve conduction.

The science of *how humans move* is called kinesiology. Within kinesiology there are many subfields, including one known as biomechanics. Biomechanics is the study of Newtonian physics (things like gravity, pressure, and friction) applied to living tissues. My personal area of study is the biomechanics of disease and injury, and I am dedicated to teaching the basic principles of physical science to people just like you, for the purpose of preventing and reversing damage to the human body.

This book is also about something bigger than your feet (even if you have really big feet). This book will also talk about ailments north of the ankles that are being influenced by the state of your feet—ailments created where other body parts are responding to the impact of your footwear. Because of the way our health care system is segmented, experts of the feet don't typically talk to the experts of the spine or experts of the nervous system. Medical experts are thoroughly trained in the biological sciences as opposed to the physical sciences; since we all look for solutions using what's in our own tool bag, those who research human ailments tend to look for solutions in chemistry (pharmaceuticals) or genetics.

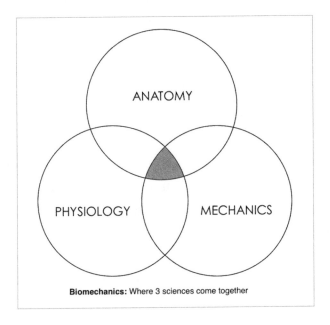

Biomechanics: Where 3 sciences come together

From the biomechanical field, research on changes in human geometry and body positioning and how they create loading damage on tissue is only now emerging in the medical journals. The effects geometry has on physical forces like pressure, friction, and gravity have been thoroughly understood in the physical sciences for hundreds of years. Mathematical proofs, along with the basic laws of Newtonian physics, apply as much to the human body as to any other physical structure in our universe. The more one understands the anatomical structures and physiological processes that drive human tissue regeneration, the clearer the picture becomes. This book will explain the mechanics of how common foot ailments develop in response to the geometrical changes footwear places on the human body. While the solutions to these ailments may seem simple, keep in mind the science behind the solutions is as consistent as gravity itself.

Specific foot ailments run the gamut, but in general, a foot ailment of any kind interferes with the ability of the entire body to function. There is hardly a human movement that does not involve the feet. No matter the current condition of your feet, you will find some piece of information in this book that will improve *how you move*, and in return, improve *how you feel*.

On a final note, while the information in this book applies equally to men (the same mechanical laws apply to their feet), I have chosen to write this book especially for women. There are several reasons behind my decision, the primary one being that women tend to make much, much poorer choices about footwear than men do. They also tend to be the purchaser of footwear for both themselves and their families. Educating the Footwear Goddess of the family on foot care and footwear physics can save an entire family of feet in one book.

A word of caution: this book is not a substitute for professional care but rather a manual on how things work in your feet, and how to alter the habits that may be contributing to your problem. Human tissue is phenomenal stuff. When you make small changes in your movement patterns, you nudge yourself down a new physiological path. The body works to tear down old or underused tissue every day, and builds up tissues that are in greatest demand. The body continuously adapts to whatever you are doing *now*.

Changing your habits will change your life!

CHAPTER 1

Welcome to ... Your Foot

"He shifted his weight from foot to foot, but it was equally uncomfortable on each."

—Douglas Adams

First, let me congratulate you. Picking up this book is the first step toward improving the health of your feet, knees, hips, pelvis, spine, and bones. This book contains information that has never been organized for public consumption. Most of what you are about to read was dredged up from the depths of academic research as part of my master's thesis. I designed most of the exercise protocol not only to make the foot healthy but also to optimize how the foot works with all of the other tissues in the body. At my alignment center in California, The Restorative Exercise Institute, many people have been successful in repairing their own feet by learning and following these exercises. Some have shared their stories in this book to help motivate and inspire you and to illustrate that the solution really can be this simple.

There are three likely reasons this book has called out to you:

1. You have feet.
2. You love the human body, preventive medicine, and anything to do with health.
3. As you are reading this, you have an aching, stabbing soreness, swelling, stiffening, bunion-ing, smashing, cramping, and/or a limping sensation in your feet. You also have a closet of very cute shoes, along with a vague notion that the two may be related. (Here's a hint: you're right.)

You have had your feet since birth. You've had them in your mouth, you've had them stepped on, and you have definitely had them squished into what seemed like a good fashion choice at the time. But chances are that you have no idea of the complex machinery living below the ankles. While you have about 200 bones in your entire body, 25 percent of them reside from the ankles down! The same goes for your muscles—a quarter of all the muscles and motor nerves in your body are dedicated to your feet. All of these movable parts, and yet I bet you don't have the same ability to move your feet as you do your fingers, despite being born with that potential!

A keen student of the natural sciences, Leonardo da Vinci referred to the foot as the most complex piece of machinery ever designed. Don't let this statement mislead you, however, into thinking that understanding your anatomy is over your head. While the function of the foot is fantastically detailed, you will be amazed at how easy it is to navigate your way around a complicated area when you have a map. Wait, did you not get your map to the foot? Well, here it is!

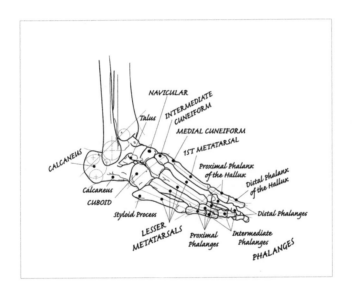

Just kidding.

You probably don't need to know this much anatomy in order to successfully steer yourself to healthier feet. That being said, you probably need to know a little bit more than this:

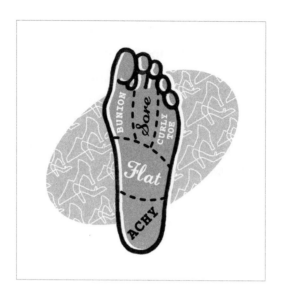

When it comes down to it, most of us know more about our cars than our bodies. Knowing the basics of automobile maintenance and performance parameters can significantly reduce the wear and tear on your car; the same goes for your anatomical parts.

To make significant headway toward healthy feet, you don't have to know the name of every single bone, muscle, tendon, and ligament that you can find in your feet, but you should know the general landscape and some basic terms.

In addition, a little information goes a long way when it comes to your ability to self-assess your ranges of motion, giving you an objective measure for your level of foot health. Knowing the correct anatomical terms will also help you to communicate with more self-empowerment should you need to make a medical appointment. As a five-year-old, I'd have to point to a body location when the doctor asked, "Where does it hurt?" It's kind of embarrassing when you have to do the same thing as a thirty-, forty-, or sixty-year-old. With the number of baby boomers on the rise, and the steadily declining state of health across the country, the time has come to take more responsibility for our own personal health. Of course, if you are reading this book, you have already accepted that responsibility. Good for you!

THE HISTORY OF FEET

Feet and man go back a long way. In fact, they go back all the way, right to the beginning. They grew up together, and evolved together, for hundreds of thousands of years before any shoes showed up on the scene. In the modern world, shoes have served to protect our living tissue from the unnatural surfaces that generate excessive forces, both at the surface (skin), and below it (bone). The increase of man-made debris has also created safety issues while walking barefoot through natural environments. Stemming from pre-antibiotic days when foot puncture could be catastrophic even for even a healthy person, footwear gradually evolved from light surface protection to fully engineered full-body stabilizers like the hiking boot. Very recently a whole new category of footwear—healthy shoes—has emerged, along with myriad enticing claims about how a particular shoe design can increase health or fitness levels by doing nothing more than wearing them.

Footwear evolution has achieved a level of almost complete protection of the tissue from the environment. The protection of the foot has steadily become the encasing of the foot, usually by materials more rigid than the feet themselves. In other words, what da Vinci called "a masterpiece of engineering," a machine whose refined design evolved over millennia, is now stuck in one of your shoes. When an engineer begins making repairs or modifications to any machine—whether made of metal or organic tissue—the engineer has to ask the question: what else might this change affect?

A biomechanist, looking at the mechanics of the human body, will ask a similar question: for all of the benefit that protective footwear may bring, what else might it affect?

Consider all of the bones and muscles that make up and control your hands and fingers, and how many wonderfully unique ways you can move them. The ability to type, play the piano, conduct surgeries on microscopic tissue, and even the ability to pluck your eyebrows are all a result of learning how to use the muscles in your hands, and keeping them limber through regular use. Now imagine that when you were two years old, someone placed stiff, tight leather mittens over your hands, lumping all of the bones together, every day, from morning to night. Your body would adapt to the situation, learning how to use the muscles of the forearms and the joints of the wrist to a greater extent. You would learn to use the outside edge of your hand as one "finger" and train the digits to all work as one body part. This way of using your hands would be completely normal to you, as that is the way it would always have been.

Now ponder this: the intricate design of your feet indicates the potential for them to be about as dexterous as your hands. Really! But the act of wearing shoes every day has created a mitten-hand situation in your feet—and you didn't even know it! We have weak, underdeveloped muscles within the foot and have placed large loads on the muscles of the lower leg, on the joints in the foot, and on passive tissues (those that cannot adapt strength) like the fascial systems and ligaments of the foot.

The good news is, by learning a bit more about your foot-machines, you can restore a lot of lost function and start the repair process right away. As long as your feet contain living tissue, they can change, grow, and improve, no matter what they've been doing (or not doing) up to this point!

Anatomy Lesson One: Your toes are separate structures from your feet for a reason.

Typically when we think of the feet, we include everything from the ankle down. Lumping this whole area together in our minds has the end result of lumping all the tissues together in our using patterns. Each toe, just like each finger, has its own set of muscles that allow it to function independently. While there are no modern functional activities that require us to use our toes individually, there is a bigger purpose for being wired this way. Every muscle has its own nerve supply that, when activated, keeps that area of the body well nourished. While writing with our toes is not required for daily living (thank goodness—my penmanship is bad enough as it is!), being able to generate these movements is required for optimal health in that area.

Anatomy Lesson Two: Your toes should move separately from your feet.

Many people, especially those with chronic foot issues, cannot lift their toes without lifting their foot when standing. Go ahead and try this. Stand up (it's okay, you can take the book with you), kick your shoes off, and see if you can isolate the muscles in your toes without taking the entire foot with them. If you don't get it right away, try backing your hips up so your weight is over your heels, and keep practicing. You'll be surprised how quickly your toes may go from zero to some movement with a little bit of diligence.

Anatomy Lesson Three: Your toes should move separately from each other.

Look at all of the unique motions you can create with your fingers, lifting them one or two at a time, playing a piano, or even typing. We have the same potential in our feet as we do our hands, but we have neglected these muscle groups for our entire lives, and we are left with stiff tissues, weak and atrophied muscles, and degenerating joints in the feet. No wonder they hurt! If you had fun with the last exercise, you're going to love this one. Try lifting your toes individually, without bringing along the rest of the gang. I suggest starting with your big toe (see page 107 for an illustration of this motion).

Don't worry if you can't do it now. You will learn eventually, with practice. In fact, many people who are without arms or hands train their feet to complete daily tasks—from diapering a baby, to writing, to playing the piano. All of the pulleys, levers, and electrical equipment are in place—we just have to learn how to use them.

Anatomy Lesson Four: The front half of your foot should move separately from the back half.

Now that I've told you your toes are separate structures, keep in mind that the foot is not just one giant, fixed bone, but is made up of twenty-six bones and thirty-three joints! The primary reason our body even has joints is to allow for fluidity while moving. Could you imagine how hard it would be to use your arms or legs if your elbows or knees were missing? Your movements would be extremely rigid and stiff! The same goes for your foot: the less you use the many small joints within your foot by moving it in unique and novel ways, the less fluid control you have over stabilizing your body's weight. Stabilizing your body's weight means carrying it over the most resilient part of the foot (i.e., the heel) while walking, instead of letting your body's mass crush and strain the more delicate sets of ligaments and bones.

Wondering what happened to the arch of your foot? Believe it or not, there is no anatomical "part" that holds the arches of the feet. The arch is merely a shape created by what the muscles and bones are doing. If this area of your foot is giving you problems, you still need to address both the strength and flexibility of the feet. Whether completely missing, or high and stiff, the exercise prescription is the same.

The Fit Feet exercises shown later in this book will help you develop strength and mobility in all the right places.

FOOT MUSCLES

It is important to understand that every muscle has its very own nerve supply. When you underuse any of the muscles in the body, the communication between the nerves and the muscles decreases, which results in a decrease in the health of both tissues. The inverse is also true: increasing the use of every individual muscle can improve the health of both muscle and nerve tissues by increasing circulation. Increased circulation means bringing oxygen-rich blood (tissue "food") to the area and removing waste products—waste that would otherwise accumulate and accelerate tissue breakdown.

The nerves that are responsible for moving the foot muscles originate from the lower parts of your spinal column. Traveling from your spine all the way to your feet, these nerves are some of the longest in your entire body.

The muscles of the feet are put into two groups, extrinsic and intrinsic. Extrinsic muscles are those with one end residing within the foot, and the other end residing somewhere outside of the foot. The muscles of your calves are examples of extrinsic foot muscles. These muscles move the foot around, but are not contained completely within the foot.

Intrinsic muscles are those muscles that are contained completely within the foot. These muscles are much smaller, and they are responsible for tiny, controlling movements of the many joints in the foot. An example of an intrinsic foot muscle would be the abductor digiti minimi, the muscle that moves the little toe out and away from the rest of the foot. Ever heard of it? I didn't think so.

ALL ABOUT YOUR PIGGIES

- In the medical community, the toes are numbered outward, from the big toe (Toe #1) to the pinky toe (Toe #5).
- The bones in the toes are called foot phalanges (fa-LAN-gees).
- There are three phalanges in each toe except for the big toe, which has only two. This gives the smaller toes the ability to curl better than Toe #1.

If we think back to the example of covering our hands with leather mittens, it would be the intrinsic muscles that would become underdeveloped due to lack of fine movements. The extrinsic muscles would have to work more to compensate for the lack of help. This is what's going on with our feet. Ideally, the intrinsic muscles work in coordination with the extrinsic muscles to move the toes by themselves, optimize the shape and position of the foot arch, and keep the nerve-muscle relationships of the foot optimized.

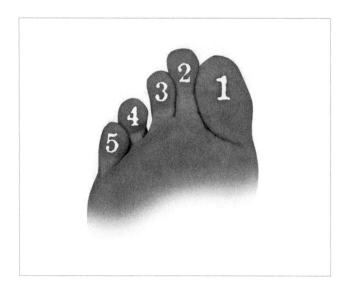

FAST PHALANGE FACTS

TOE #1: *Hallux* is the Latin word for the big toe. It was derived from the Greek verb meaning "to spring" or "to leap." The tip of the big toe is the last part of your body to leave the ground after your pelvis (where your center of mass is) vaults into your next step.

TOE #2: The second toe, also called the index or long toe, can be the same length or sometimes longer than the big toe. This condition is typically referred to as a Morton's toe. Oftentimes people will experience pain in this toe and be told that the longer toe is the problem. While a long second phalange will change the way the bones in the foot are loaded, damage to this area is caused not just by the toe itself, but by a particular gait pattern coupled with the extra-long appendage. If you are dealing with pain and have a Morton's toe, you can change the mechanics of how you move to decrease the pain!

TOE #3: Ask most Americans, and they'll tell you that this little piggy, the "middle toe," had roast beef. To the British, who are not renowned for their cuisine, this little piggy typically has bread and butter. Sad. Those with webbed toes (a not-that-uncommon condition called syndactyly) will usually experience a tighter bond between the second and third digit together. Here's a fun fact: some famous folks with webbed toes include Dan Aykroyd, Ashton Kutcher, and Joseph Stalin.

TOE #4: The fourth toe doesn't have a special name. Maybe that's why people wear toe rings, just to boost this toe's self-esteem. This toe does have a greater risk for brachymetatarsia ("brachy"—short; "metatarsals"—bones in the foot), a bone that stops growing at a young age. Many people with a shortened fourth toe may notice some of the surrounding toes moving underneath, leading to painful walking patterns and "rubbing injuries" like corns and calluses.

Even though I have all my toes, I have been walking on only four toes ever since I was little.

My next-to-pinky toe stopped growing at a certain age in my childhood, and that shorter toe has made it hard to find shoes that fit. Shoes either had to have lots of space in the front because the short toe sticks up (the pinky toe has curled underneath that toe to support it), or go high enough that they don't rub that toe and make it sore. Can you imagine cramming that toe into heels and walking without it hurting? Not a good idea, of course, but I have done it anyway, since high school! Your exercises and Earth brand's wide toe box has helped me so much to be able to spread my toes now and the shoes don't rub the top of my toe next to my pinky toe and make it sore. No more sore and aching feet! I am forever grateful!

—LANENE W.

TOE #5: This little guy got the cutest name of all: pinky. Typically the smallest of the toes, this little guy, unable to defend itself against fashionable footwear, is often greatly displaced when wearing your favorite pair of shoes and develops a corn as a response to the extra pressure or friction from the tight fit.

CORNEUM, CORNS, AND CALLUSES, OH MY!

There are lots of visual signs you can learn to read that give you insight into how you use your body. Corns and calluses are actually very clear visual signals that your body is experiencing excessive pressure or friction.

Have you ever wondered what a corn is, or how it got its name?

The top layer of your skin is made of dead cells and is called the *Stratum corneum*. Corneum is derived from the Latin word for "horned," as this layer is the oldest and "hardest" of the five layers that make up the outer layer of your skin.

The normal physiological response to mechanical irritation (increased rubbing or squeezing) is to "beef up" the area, to protect irritated skin. This thickening process is called hyperkeratosis ("hyper"—excessive; "kerat"—from the word keratin, a family of structural proteins; "osis"—the process of).

A "corn" is the small, kernel-shaped result of hyperkeratosis, which is a result of how your foot is interacting with its environment (shoe or landscape). A callus is the same thing, only more flat and broad compared to a corn. The most common place people develop a corn is along the outside of the pinky toe, although they can form wherever skin is pushing into something foreign. Calluses are typically found on the sole of the foot, where pressure is the greatest.

An interesting note: calluses are actually areas of the skin that have much better circulation than other areas. What makes a callus uncomfortable is due to the fact that it is only a small area of thicker skin. This small patch of "health" becomes like a rock in a shoe (or a pea under a mattress if you're a princess).

The optimal way to get super-regenerating skin would be to allow our foot to interact with the natural outside-shoe world over a lifetime, prompting a slow adaptation in foot skin thickness over that lifetime, giving us a much better ability to cope with the sensations caused by walking barefoot.

Key Points, Chapter One

1. The anatomy of the foot indicates that our feet have the potential to move in much more complex ways then we actually use them.

2. Allowing the complex machinery of the foot to go unused or underused allows muscles to atrophy.

3. Most foot problems are a result of disuse, combined with overloading the underused tissue.

4. The muscles in your feet are exactly the same as the muscles in the rest of the body; they respond and adapt to regular use and specific exercise.

5. Retraining the muscles in the feet can increase the regeneration of the tissue that lives there, which can decrease disease and increase the overall health of your feet.

CHAPTER 2

Where Do *Your* Feet Stand?

"People are crying up the rich and variegated plumage of the peacock, and he is himself blushing at the sight of his ugly feet."

—Sa'di

O nce you have the basics of the anatomy of both the foot and footwear, you can begin to get objective about your own body. Don't worry, you aren't the only person who cringes at the thought of baring it all, especially when it comes to your feet. Before we start poking and prodding and measuring and quantifying your tootsies, you will need to remove the mask. And by mask, I mean your shoes. And yes, the socks have to come off, too. You can't tell what your feet are doing until you can see them—clearly.

Now that you know a little more about your anatomy, it's time to get scientific and do some data collection. I'm going to walk you step-by-step through parts of your foot that you didn't even know you had! I've even included images and tasks to help you evaluate what is happening below your ankles.

We often forget, while cringing at the appearance of our feet (or any body part, for that matter), that how our feet look is simply a reflection of how we have been using them. Lumps and bumps, calluses and dry patches, bone spurs, inflamed nerves, and even fractures are simply the result of what we have done with our feet. Undoubtedly genetics are a contributing factor, as various bone lengths and certain skin qualities increase the risk for certain ailments. Most genetic factors, however, are not diseases in themselves. Genes are simply qualities of human tissue that, when combined with particular habits or environmental conditions, might result in chronic pain or injury. Since you can't do much about your genetics, you need to stop mistreating your feet! And developing good habits is the best way available to ensure the long-term health of your feet.

The good news is this: the current state of your feet is influenced by habits that are easy to identify and modify. The two habits we have that most significantly impact the structure of the foot's tissues are the shoes we wear, and the way we use our feet to move ourselves around. Footwear, as you will continue to learn, is responsible for a host of problems that directly contribute to foot pain and tissue degeneration. You have total control over what is in your closet, so footwear is really the easiest thing to change. When it comes to walking, you'll have to start paying a little more attention to your body in order make lasting changes, but the payoff is worth it.

If you are reading this book, you have probably been walking for longer than you can remember. Done by just about everyone, every day, few consider how they walk. They just do it. Yet your gait pattern has a similar effect on your body, just like proper wheel alignment affects your car. And in this case, your feet are the best indication of where your foot "wheels" are pointing—and how many miles they have left!

NOBODY WALKS EXACTLY LIKE YOU

Your particular gait pattern (which is a fancy way of saying the way you walk) is an extremely complex, whole-body coordination system that is completely unique to you. Walking patterns are very similar to talking patterns. In the same way that the speaking accent you have is similar to that of your parents, the first influence on your "walking accent" was the way others around you moved. Like all animals, humans learn a lot about movement through observation. This is also why so many of us end up walking in a manner similar to our parents. After the initial pattern is set, your walking style is further enhanced by other activities you have done with regularity. Ballet dancers tend to develop a "ballerina turnout" even after they've left dance class. Those with military training keep the "at attention" feet long after anyone is checking. Walking with chronic pain, or even limping along after an injury—especially after a stint on crutches—can leave a person with an altered pattern that goes unnoticed (and thus uncorrected). And finally, many add a bit of their own walking "flair." These are little postural adjustments of choice. We mimic the style of people we admire, or demonstrate an attitude or emotion we'd like to convey via body language.

All of these influence the position of our joints (including our foot joints!) and eventually, our alignment becomes a habit.

Your gait pattern can be measured and quantified with a lot of expensive and highly sophisticated biomechanical equipment. But here's a secret: you can also just look down to see what your feet are doing. This is a low-tech evaluation for sure, but still a highly effective way to see how you are moving. One interesting biomechanical tidbit about your body is that the position you have learned to acquire in order to balance while walking is the same alignment you maintain while standing. Analyzing your stance is easier when first starting—trying to walk and analyze your gait can be a bit challenging!

WHAT SHOULD YOUR FOOT BE DOING?

As your body moves through each stride, many things are happening at the same time. The foot, in particular, should have four distinct positions it passes through with each step! These positions are:

1. Heel strike—only the heel is planted on the floor.
2. Foot flat—the front of the foot comes down to join the heel and now the entire foot is on the ground.
3. Heel off—the heel leaves, but the front of the foot remains.
4. Toe off—the straggling forefoot and toes finally leave the ground and move toward another step!

In order for the foot to achieve each of these four specific points, the lower leg, foot, and toes have to be mobile enough to allow it. Tight calves, stiff ankles, and inflexible foot joints make this more difficult, and some of the points may be missed occasionally, or left out entirely! The "senior shuffle" is a walking pattern that bypasses most of these points, with the walker simply sliding a flat foot along the ground, or raising it minimally. In addition to the fact that this low-quality gait pattern is damaging to the feet, it also increases the risk for tripping, since it greatly reduces the clearance the foot has over rogue objects like cords and cracks in the sidewalk!

TAKE A LOOK

The best way to start off your foot analysis is to examine the position of your feet while standing with bare feet, in a stance that is your normal, comfortable, everyday stance. I suggest you don't look at your feet until you have taken a lap around your room, looking straight ahead. Now stop, and settle into your comfortable stance without looking.

Look down and take a moment to observe your stance.

First, check for symmetry. Are both feet doing exactly the same thing, or is one foot turned out more than the other?

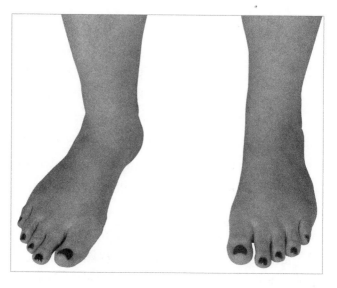

Would you drive a car with wheels aligned like this?

Symmetry is just as important to maintain in the smaller segments of the body as it is when considering whole-body posture. As in any machine, working some parts harder than others results in different wear patterns than the manufacturer probably considered. In the foot, even wear is the goal; over- or underloading can cause skin patches that differ in resilience, bones that are reinforced to take greater loads than they should, and muscles that are used more or less frequently than what is optimal. These are all considered ailments, but they are just normal tissue changes based on use patterns. These problems can be corrected.

Though your body requires symmetrical use to function optimally, we tend to practice one-sided motions in our modern culture, like driving, writing, or dominant-sided sports. These activities use one side of the body more than the other, and this affects how the musculature develops. These muscle patterns, in turn, can pull on our bones, even to the point of displacing them!

There are other things that influence symmetry as well; an injury, for example, can cause us to shift our weight to the uninjured side to allow us to keep functioning while we're healing. All too often, however, a freshly healed person will fail to return to a more symmetrical pattern of movement. Or, perhaps when learning how to walk, you mimicked the nonsymmetrical pattern of someone in your household. No matter the reason, noticing the symmetry (or lack thereof) is the first step to reconciling your gait.

Second, check out the direction your feet point. Do they look like the wheels on a car, both pointing fairly straight ahead (correct), or do they veer away from the center of your body (incorrect)?

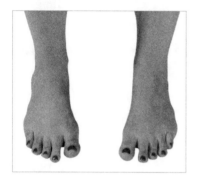
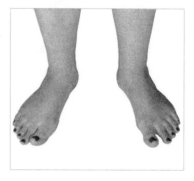

Correct   *Incorrect*

The reason your wheels point forward on the car is (obviously) to propel your car straightforward. When the alignment is off, the motion of the out-of-whack tire against the road pulls the car forward and sideways at the same time. As a driver, you try to correct the sideways pull, which takes a toll on both you and the car; as you force the car to straighten up, the tire wears prematurely. The same holds true for the non-forward-pointing foot. When the foot isn't positioned to move straightforward, the muscles in the lower leg that would normally contract are not able to do their job, and muscles that have other responsibilities are now required to participate in your particular way of walking.

The greater the turn-out of your foot, the less your foot moves through the normal heel-toe cycle, and the more it lands on the outside of your foot, rolling in toward the inside of your foot. This disrupts the normal heel-toe cycle of forward propulsion, and replaces it with an outside-to-inside cycle. Or more simply, you have a weight-bearing piece of machinery that is working in a direction it wasn't designed to handle over the long term.

When we look at the direction a foot is headed, sometimes we are really only looking at the toes. The toes seem to be pointing straight ahead, so that must mean the foot is, too, right? Actually, when measuring foot position, it is best to look at the outside edge of the foot—not the toes or the curved instep. Using the straight edge of a carpet or yoga mat, check to see how far the outside portion of your foot deviates from the border. Try moving the outside edge of your foot until it lines up with the straight edge of the carpet. How does that feel? Odd? Odd is okay, and probably good for your foot.

Speaking of the toes, how do they look? You can check for symmetry in the individual bones, comparing those on the right foot to those on the left. Toes, even though they are pretty small pieces of machinery, possess the ability to do a whole lot of interesting movements. They can move to the right or left. They can lift up off of the floor, curl down into the sand, and they can twist and turn—especially if your gait is less than optimal.

A NOTE ON TURN-OUT

Many experts will argue that there is a natural turn-out to the foot. This data comes from measuring a large population of people and making measurements of commonly found postural positions. It is true that reviewing data in this way will show that almost everyone in our population does, in fact, have a slight turn-out to the foot. That, however, does not prove that there is a natural turn-out to the foot, only that most of us have one.

If you consider the cultural habits most western Europeans have shared for the last few hundred years, you will see two common trends: military training and ballet. Each of these traditions has a strong, enforced postural component. The "turned-out feet with heels together" posture is culturally inspired, as opposed to naturally formed (meaning "from nature"). Yet, because a large quantity of our recent ancestors have been exposed to this training, this posture begins to engrain itself into what is "normal"—as quantified by how the majority of us stand. "Normal," "common," and "regular" are very different from "natural."

Modern exercise protocols that use dance as a platform tend to portray this turn-out as actual proper alignment, as opposed to proper alignment specifically for dance.

We learn movement from our elders, teachers, and movement therapists, and nearly everyone is teaching turn-out, either directly or indirectly. Yet, when you actually examine the complex engineering of the toes, foot, joints, inner foot, and lower leg musculature, the position of the foot and ankle best suited to the long-term function of all of the tissues is aimed straight ahead.

Even if data is collected in a scientific manner, it does not mean the conclusions are necessarily valid. Think of the data collected for today's populations—weight, fitness level, hamstring flexibility, etc. Our physical states—even our personal, slow-to-change skeletal positions—are still a direct result of user habit. I, for one, would never want textbooks of the future referencing the obesity statistics of today's population as "natural" or "normal" in any way!

After walking with an excessive turn-out for a long period of time, turning your dogs straight ahead will likely result in you feeling more turned-in. Of course, that's because your feet are more turned-in. You're not turned-in too much (you can use the outside edge of the foot as a gauge), but probably a lot more than you were before. And now that your feet are pointing forward, your toes may be curving in toward the center line of your body. That's okay, too.

CONTINUED ON NEXT PAGE...

CONTINUED ...

They've been like that for a while, you just probably never noticed. If you have been walking with
your feet turned-out for a long time, your toes may
have realigned themselves to stay pointing ahead,
even though the foot itself is turned-out. As you
strengthen the neglected muscles in the toes (see
pages 107–113), you can improve the muscular tone
and impact their position as well.

Toes without much healthy musculature really get
pushed around by the way you use your feet. Without well-
developed muscles to keep them stable, toes can end up in
each other's space, creating a traffic jam of sorts. When one
toe gets pulled too far in one direction, it ends up, literally,
on top of your other toes. This is usually blamed on joint
instability, but keep in mind, the first line of joint stability is
the muscle system. Neglect exercising those little inner-foot
muscles, and you will end up with side stepping toes!

This is also a good time to see if you have any hammertoes. These toes buckle up above the others, and can rub on
the inside of your shoe, creating redness, soreness, or eventually a corn.

Become a Photo Detective
ACTIVITY BOX

Our major walking and postural patterns were set very early on, as we learned to move by mimicking those around us. The moral of the story is this: the state of your physical body is the sum total of *how you have used it*. But you don't have to take my word for it—if you've got photos, you can be your own alignment detective!

Find the earliest photos of yourself that allow you to pay special attention to your feet. In those first-year baby photos, how do your feet look? Use both the symmetry and position-evaluating skills you have just acquired to create an alignment timeline. Here is an example from my personal collection:

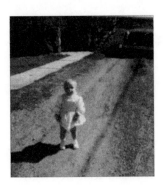

Here I am at about one year old. Check out my foot position; looking pretty straight at this point.

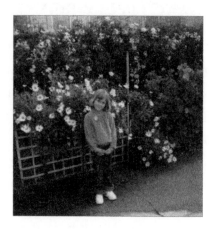

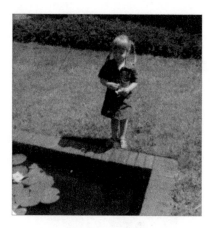

In all of my pictures taken between ages three and four, you can see that my right foot has started turning out.

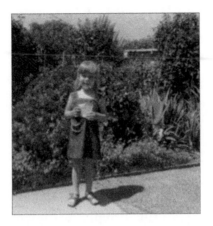

This is a pattern of standing (and walking) that stays with me for years, as I use the pictures to investigate my habit history.

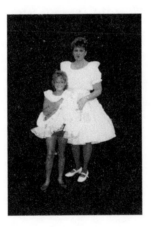

These pictures of my mom and me (who doesn't love a good petticoat picture?) show that someone else in the family has the same habit. Aha!

My detective work here is done!

Key Points, Chapter 2

1. Genetic factors play a role in disease, but the real culprit in many chronic conditions is *how* we use the tissue we are given.
2. Two easily modifiable habits are the shoes we select and the way we walk.
3. Our pattern of walking is a result of observing how others walked while we learned to walk, in addition to dance, sport, or military training, and our personal choice of "style."
4. Expensive equipment can evaluate our gait pattern, but we can just check it out in the mirror to make basic adjustments—for free!

CHAPTER 3

The Foot Bone *Is* Connected to the Hip Bone

"Toe bone connected to the foot bone
"Foot bone connected to the leg bone
"Leg bone connected to the knee bone..."
—"Dem Bones"

I n addition to becoming more aware of where your feet are pointing when walking, there are other parts of the body that affect what is happening to your feet. Because the feet carry the weight of the body, every body part can affect the overall loading on your feet. Trying to figure out how each of your body parts is stacked over your feet can take a lot of mathematical analysis. For the sake of time, let us identify just one of your body parts that has a heavy influence on the health of your feet—your pelvis.

The pelvis is important to foot heath because it is essentially your *center of mass*. This means that wherever your pelvis is, so is the bulk of your weight. Ideally, your body segments stack up in a straight line from your ankles all the way to the top of your head. Yet most of us walk around with our hips out forward of our feet, creating a motion that is less like walking, and more like falling.

Holding your pelvis out in front of you creates all sorts of unwanted consequences throughout the body, especially the feet. A forward pelvis positions your weight right over the front of the feet, loading the small bones and tissues of the forefoot. The densest structure of the foot is in the back of the foot; the large heel bone is much better equipped for long-term weight-bearing. Designed to take the bulk of your weight, the heel can only do this job if you adjust the rest of your body back where it belongs.

YOUR "PELVIS POSTURE"

Find your pelvis. When you put your hands on your hips, you are essentially placing them on your pelvis, just above the actual hip joints. When you are standing, your weight should line up vertically from your ankles to your knees and hips.

We all have an idea that good posture means standing up straight, but what often happens is that instead of getting all major joint points stacked up vertically (correct), we end up with an exaggerated posture (incorrect) that is no longer vertical.

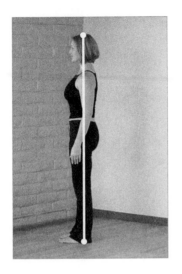 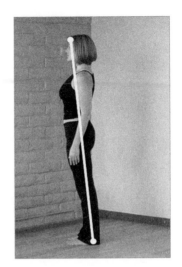

Correct   *Incorrect*

When we *think* of "good posture" we often *think* "shoulders back," but when we *do* "good posture," often we're not really pulling our arms back as much as we are pushing our pelvis forward. Unfortunately for our feet, *hips forward* has become the new *shoulders back*. I realize this doesn't seem like a big deal to most people, but from a mechanical perspective, when your alignment—your vertical stacking—is altered significantly, the resulting geometry changes the flow to and loading on various tissue.

Keeping the pelvis stacked correctly is an essential part of foot health. Drawing a vertical line down from the center of mass clearly shows the difference in weight placement, which is over the front of the feet when the pelvis is too far forward.

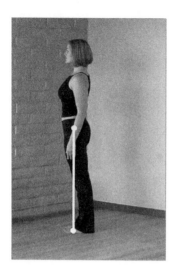 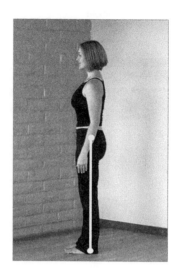

On the left, the burden is obviously great on the front of the feet, overloading tiny muscles that *should* be focused on supporting the arch of the feet—not the weight of the body. This weight on the front of the feet can also be a contributing factor to plantar fasciitis, hammertoes, metatarsalgia (pain in the base of the toes), and neuropathy. Stacking your weight over the back of your feet allows the weight to be supported by your skeleton, from hips to heels.

ARE YOU WEIGHT-BEARING?

Everyone reading this book has either experienced bone loss firsthand, or knows someone who has been told of decreasing bone mineral density somewhere in their skeleton. Osteoporosis has become a national health care crisis as the affliction rate is not only increasing, but increasing in younger and younger populations. But where does it come from? The phenomenon of bone mineral loss has many components—nutrition, hormones, genes, and *alignment*. Wait, did I say alignment? Absolutely!

Two main reasons the major axis of the body should form a vertical line is to minimize forces that cause joint degeneration (ankles, knees, hips, lumbar, and thoracic spine), and to maximize structural support (weight over the dense heel bones instead of over plantar fascia and forefeet). Vertical positioning also places the weight of the upper body directly over the pelvis, which makes the hip joints fully *weight-bearing*.

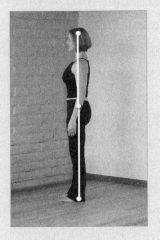 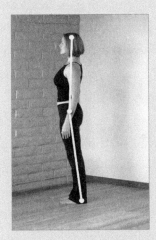

More weight-bearing   *Less weight-bearing*

CONTINUED ON NEXT PAGE...

CONTINUED ...

Misunderstanding the meaning of "weight-bearing," many people are trying to increase the loading of their bones by adding hand weights to their daily walks and upping the resistance on the machines at the gym. However, to be weight-bearing, the key is to line up your body with the force that makes "weight," which is the vertical force of gravity.

To better understand this, let us take a look at how bone regeneration works. When a bone is loaded (meaning the force of weight is put on it), it responds by maintaining enough structural strength to support that weight. Bone strength comes from bone minerals. Now here's the clincher: the creator of "weight" is gravity—and gravity is a force that only works in the perpendicular or vertical direction. This means that bones are loaded under your full body weight only when they are stacked vertically. No extra weight is really needed to maintain bone density—your body weight loaded on your vertical bones should be good enough to keep maximal bone density. But when you have a positive heel underneath your ankle with every step (and so many of us have had a positive heel underneath our feet for practically our entire lives), your bones are pitched forward and no longer vertical, decreasing the weight placed on the bones of your hips, and decreasing the signal to build bone in that area. The femoral neck, the part of the hip most sensitive to bone loss, is simply not receiving the osteogenic (bone-building) message, and all because of your footwear choice. Ouch!

ALIGNMENT—THE QUICK FIX

Get your weight back where it belongs! It's easy, fast, and free. You may also notice that adjusting your weight off of your toes and onto your heels is just about impossible when wearing a positive-heeled shoe. Shoes with *any* heel automatically prevent vertical alignment because of the angular changes created at the ankle.

When barefoot, try backing your hips up, getting your weight far enough back to lift your toes off the ground. Now you have a sense of your weight being over your heels!

Once you learn to evaluate posture using objective markers (like a vertical line), physical forces like loading and joint torque are easier to understand. A line that is not vertical allows anyone with a mechanical eye to "see" the forward lean, which causes damage to structures due to overloading, as in the feet, or underloading, as in the bones of the hips.

BACK PAIN BONUS

The back pain caused by the positive heel is most likely due to the pelvic changes created by footwear. The forward thrust of the hips can couple with the altered tilt of the pelvis needed to deal with the geometrical changes in the body. The result can be an increase in the pressure on the sacroiliac joint, as well as a shift in the loading patterns of the lower spine.

If, in addition to foot issues, you notice back pain, or your health care provider has diagnosed you with an ailment of the lower back, finding out you are a pelvis thruster may provide you with a clue to help you decrease the misloading of this area.

Backing your hips up until they make a vertical line with the knees and ankles will feel like you're sticking your bum out. Get objective about it first. What you "feel" and what "is" are two different things. There's nothing like a sideways view in a full-length mirror to help you see where your body parts actually are. And start paying attention to how your body feels when aligned and barefoot compared with when wearing a shoe with a heel. The more mindful you are about your body, the more you will start to feel different tissue squishing into position when you slip something onto your feet!

> *I was diagnosed with a bone spur on the top of my foot at the base of the big toe. It was very painful, red, and swollen and limited my walking because it hurt all the time. I went to the podiatrist for his input and he told me the pain would "continue to intensify until a year from now I would be begging him to do surgery to correct it."*

I started making changes with my stance and walking pattern, the feet straight ahead was very helpful as was putting the weight on my heels and changing all of my shoes to flats or negative heels. It wasn't long before my pain and the redness went away and with no swelling, I was able to enjoy walking again pain free. Well, I have continued to follow your alignment guidelines and still no pain after nine months! It even seems to be a bit smaller!

—DIANE L., Physical Therapist

Key Points, Chapter 3

1. Your pelvis can be another factor in chronic foot ailments, as its position can load the tissue in the incorrect places, i.e., the front of the feet, as opposed to the more bone-dense areas of the heels and ankles.

2. Your pelvic placement is a result of your posture—thrusting your hips forward can be a mindless habit.

3. Your pelvic placement may also be a result of your compensatory mechanisms for coping with the positive-heel aspect of footwear.

4. You cannot get your pelvis off the front of your feet without getting out of positive-heeled shoes.

CHAPTER 4

Take a Stand Against Your Mother's Bunion!

"Even if genotype is the most important causal factor, in practice it is irrelevant, as it is impossible to modify one's inheritance but easy to improve footwear."

—I.B. Shine, M.D.

I was recently watching a popular doctor-hosted daytime talk show when I heard the host inform his millions of viewers that bunions were genetic. I almost fell out of my chair.

Very common in women, the bunion has been perpetuated as an unpreventable condition, stored in your genetic code, just waiting to pop out and make walking painful and wearing shoes difficult. This is not the case.

Let's talk about bunions. The term bunion possibly comes from the Greek language, meaning "small hill, mound, or heap." Or, it may come from the Latin word *bunio*, meaning "enlargement"—who knows? The development of a bunion is usually a response to unnatural loading occurring along the joints of the *hallux*, which, as you'll remember, is the Latin word for the big toe. Using the foot in a manner that is inconsistent with its design creates repetitive rotations that shouldn't be there. These constant (and sometimes tiny) twists in a walking pattern end up distorting bones and joints, which increase joint-loading, friction, and finally, swelling.

A bunion is essentially an increase in tissue development or swelling along the medial border (the side closest to the midline of your body) of the big toe, in response to how the bones operate while walking. This swelling of the bone and soft tissue decreases the joint range of motion until the *hallux* is unable to point straight ahead or spread out away from the other toes. Over time, as bone develops, the joint swelling becomes joint hardening. The *hallux* becomes fairly stuck, pointing toward the pinky toe. This toe-joint position is called *hallux valgus*. After a while, the big toe can be pulled so forcefully toward the pinky toe that it becomes almost perpendicular to the other toes. Not only does *hallux valgus* reduce the function of the foot but it can also be very uncomfortable to walk on, especially if the tissues on the side of the joint have developed a full-fledged bunion.

The incidence rate of bunions is hard to quantify, but depending on what study you read, the rates range from 0.9 percent of total population, 28.4 percent of adults, and as high as 74 percent in elderly populations. While the numbers tend to vary based on how the data is collected, the common themes in the literature demonstrate that bunions happen most frequently in women and in older populations.

For those of you looking down at your bunions, and imagining how your mother's bunions looked similar, it is easy to think, "Ah yes, my bunions are indeed genetic." But there is one thing to consider about the data collected by researchers—the population being researched. In the case of bunion research, the evaluated populations in all of the various studies are typically those who have been shoe-wearing populations for anywhere from hundreds to thousands of years. Very little is known about the incidence of *hallux valgus* before people wore shoes. Doing research on "foot mechanics" has really become research on "foot mechanics of people who have always worn shoes," which is an altogether different animal when making statements about an ailment being genetic or not.

To get a much clearer picture of where this foot ailment comes from, a population of people who had never worn shoes would be ideal for a bunion study. However, a population of historically unshod people on our modern planet would be just about impossible to find.

Fortunately, there was quite a bit of data collection from various barefooted populations in the early 1900s, measuring foot and toe angles just as these cultures were starting to wear shoes. Although some of the techniques of measurement were likely more rudimentary, the values produced from these studies tend to show that in shoeless populations, the incidence of bunions occurs more naturally in about 3 percent of the population—not a rate twenty times that.

In every body, even this 3 percent, the bunion is still caused by inappropriate loading (using the joint in the wrong position). Genetics may play a role, however, by establishing the quality of an individual's collagen content in the tissues that stabilize the joint. Some people have conditions in which their collagen content is genetically proportioned differently than others. If you are thinking that you may be in this low percentage, then the collagen issue would be in all joints, not just the big toe. If you don't have such a whole-body collagen problem, your bunions are most likely caused by habits you picked up along the way.

BUT EVERYONE IN MY FAMILY HAS BUNIONS!

Before there is a bunion, there can be the long-term displacement of the big toe (any teeny-tiny toe box wearers out there?), or there can be an incorrect loading of the joint first, causing tissue growth that pushes the big toe out of the way.

The too-tight toe box is a primary contributor to the sideways motion of the big toe, along with the elevated heel, which increases the load on the front of the foot. When your feet are all squished together, the muscles between the toes pulling them together get very tight. Begin with a daily stretch of all toes, giving extra attention to the big guy (see exercises in Chapter 9). Placing your fingers between each of the toes will help restore muscle length and joint range of motion. If you have a pretty significant angle on the *hallux*, spend some time gently stretching and pulling the big toe away from the others.

FOOT POSITION

Now let us assume that you have never worn shoes that pinched your feet. In fact, let's say you've never worn shoes at all. Bunions are made in other ways, too.

As mentioned earlier, there is a large prevalence of turned-out feet. Just look around the next time you go out walking in any public place. As mentioned before, this turn-out creates an increased amount of side-to-side motion of the foot instead of the normal front-to-back motion. The sideways use of the ankle has the weight of the body rolling not off the tip of the big toe, as in normal gait, but rolling over the side of the joint, which loads the big toe incorrectly. More simply said, when the foot is turned-out, the "bunion area" of the joint presses into the ground with each step!

Remember, the side of the joint is the side. That sounds obvious, I know, but joints are designed with the same engineering laws used in building your house. The walls don't have the same weight-bearing quality as the foundation. When you walk with a turn-out, you end up walking on your joints, or "walls," instead of the foundation. Your body responds by building up these walls, which results in bony protrusions or swelling that you see on your foot as the bunion develops.

What makes bunions seem genetic is the fact that one of your parents (usually your mom) probably had them, as did her mom, and her mom's mom, which seems like too many moms for it not to be genetic. Keep in mind that out of all the things that are handed down from generation to generation, cultural input is right up there on the list with genetics. Not only are genetic hand-me-downs like tissue makeup and bone lengths and widths affecting your physical state but other habits like walking patterns and shoe choices are also influenced by our belief system. Although our beliefs are sometimes hard to change, they are much easier to alter than our DNA!

As much as you have been helping your bunions form, there are two simple things you can do right now to begin to unload your bunions and strengthen the appropriate muscle groups for keeping you off of the side of that troublesome joint.

First, stop wearing shoes with toe boxes that are too small for your feet. Even having quirky collagen doesn't mean that you will get bunions. What it means is, when you chronically push your toes together, the joint doesn't have the ability to resist your shoe habits for long. If your feet are wider than your shoes, you are damaging the big toe joints. It's as simple as that.

Second, pay attention to your foot position while walking. You don't have to become fanatical, but if you want to allow the tissue to recover from years of incorrect loading, you need to change your loading patterns. Sounds tough, but with a little mindfulness on your daily walk, you can improve the health of your feet while improving your fitness level.

Both the evidence and the laws of physical science point to the fact that the majority of bunions are self-induced through footwear choices and gait. You can see why I was flabbergasted when a medical professional announced that this foot issue is simply your destiny and beyond your control to fix. A few simple adjustments to alignment and habits can save you years of unnecessary suffering!

Key Points, Chapter 4

1. Walking with an excessive turn-out loads the big toe joint in an incorrect place, resulting in injury commonly called a bunion.
2. The heavily angled joint position of the big toe most associated with bunions is called *hallux valgus*.
3. Research in shoe-wearing populations shows the incidence of bunions to be much higher in women and older-aged populations.
4. Research on non-shoe-wearing populations shows that the natural incidence of *hallux valgus* tends to be much lower than among shoe-wearing populations—only about 3 percent.
5. Long-term wearing of tight toe boxes impacts the soft tissue responsible for stabilizing the first joint.
6. Small habit modifications (simple exercise, correct-fitting footwear, and gait alterations) can instantly impact how the toe joint loads.

CHAPTER 5

Your Shoes ... a Map

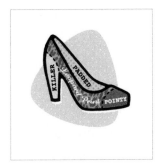

"I did not have three thousand pairs of shoes. I had one thousand and sixty."

—IMELDA MARCOS

W hew! You've made it through some tricky human anatomy and now know more about your feet than most people on the planet. Learning the parts of the shoe will be a piece of cake! Rest assured, there are only four parts of the shoe that you really need to know. With this information, you will be able to significantly increase foot health for you and your family simply by selecting the shoes best-suited to your family members' feet.

I have briefly introduced the notion that wearing footwear is an unnatural habit, and detrimental to human tissue. Yet, you might say, we have managed to compensate quite nicely as shoe-clad folks—we can walk, run, jump, compete athletically, and use our bodies quite well without really needing those smaller muscles, it seems. And we do, that is, until the day we begin to hurt.

As with any bad habit, the damage we do to our feet accumulates over time, so we don't always see the connection between what we've done and how we feel. If you are a proactive health enthusiast, you should learn all about your shoes in order to prevent ailments from arising. If you are like most of us and are motivated by current pain, you will be able to figure out which shoe styles will allow you to increase your foot health and alleviate pain. Whether you are more motivated by prevention, pain relief, or both, you need to know how to evaluate your footwear.

If you are like a lot of women, your shoes are likely purchased based on the activity for which you need them, such as sneakers for your exercise program, professional footwear for the office, or those going-out shoes that I like to call "killers." Of course, that's just the starting point! You also have such considerations as the color (red), the material (patent), and how long you can walk in them (only until you find the next chair!). You've already got your shoe shopping down to a fashion science, with equations and three-dimensional graphs. Nothing against your current system, but be prepared to involve a whole new set of variables into your science. You need a new shoe anatomy.

Each part of the shoe, in addition to acting as a lovely accessory to your outfit, has a unique way of changing the mechanics of the foot. Shoe designers, especially when it comes to athletics, performance, and "healthy" footwear, will often play with the geometry of each of these "parts" to get their shoes to do more than just decorate the feet.

Footwear design is very complex, with the engineer taking into account issues of pressure and joint instability. We're not going to get into all of the intricate parts of the shoe. All you really need to know in order to start increasing your foot health right away are the primary components that make up your shoe. Shoe anatomy is traditionally broken down into four main parts: upper, sole, toe box, and heel.

THE SOLE

The sole really is the "soul" of the shoe; it's the reason people created shoes in the first place. Designed to protect the skin from abrasions and punctures, what was originally a thin piece of animal hide has steadily progressed toward the impenetrable Fort Knox of Granny's orthopedic shoe.

The flooring of footwear ranges in terms of stiffness, thickness, squishiness, amount of contour (the lumps and bumps the manufacturer puts into the footbed), and height. Throughout recorded history, the soles of shoes have traveled the lines between healthy functionality and absurd heights, slopes, and lengths, all in the name of fashion. Each of these characteristics can affect how your feet function relative to the ground, which impacts which muscles get used in the gait cycle.

THE UPPER

The upper of a shoe is the topmost material of the shoe and is what connects your foot to the sole. Uppers range from full coverage (like a sneaker) to forefoot-only coverage (like a mule or sandal without a slingback) to a flip-flop, or as I like to call it, the string bikini of footwear.

The qualities of an upper go beyond just the amount of material covering your skin; it's also affected by what the material actually is. For example, a water shoe has a stretchy, sock-like quality that helps your foot stay in the shoe, even if much of the upper itself has been cut away. Likewise, a well-engineered Greek or Roman strappy sandal provides a good connection between the foot and the shoe without a lot of material. The crisscrossing straps adhere effectively to the foot without decreasing circulation of air across the skin of the foot, which makes this type of shoe ideal for warmer climates.

THE TOE BOX

Take a long, hard look at the front of your naked feet and toes. All of that flesh and bone has got to fit in the very front of your shoe, into what is called the toe box. Like all boxes, toe boxes come in a range of sizes—from the pointiest models of early 2000s (she who didn't participate in this fashion trend may throw the first stone!) to the wide, open front of a Greek sandal.

> *My first job in college was as a salesclerk at a department store. Women were required to wear skirts (this was back in '95), so of course I bought my first pair of heels to wear on my first day—a "sensible" brown pair with a two-inch heel. We were not allowed to sit down except during breaks, so my first eight-hour shift was excruciating! When I got home after work, I pried off my shoes and discovered that *both* of my pinky toenails were completely gone. I did not learn my lesson, though, and wore heels throughout college—and my pinky toenails didn't grow back until I got a desk job and found a nice pair of dress flats.*
>
> —LINDA

You might think foot binding is a foreign, ancient practice, but when you consider some of the toe boxes that women today are choosing to squeeze their feet into, you might not be so sure!

ALL ABOUT YOUR HEEL

Finally, and perhaps most importantly, there is the heel. This could not be a book about women's foot health without giving the high heel a little objective scrutiny.

The heel of a shoe aligns itself with the "heel" of the body. The heel is quickly becoming the most researched component of footwear, as this particular part has the ability to radically change the geometry of the human body. Just placing a little wedge under our foundation causes compensatory actions in the ankle, knee, hip, and spine, and can knock our natural gait pattern off-kilter—and it does this in an instant! The heeled shoe, believe it or not, has not always been just for women. In fact, some of the earliest versions of a high heel were worn by men, and still today, European and Latin shoe designers often use a lofty heel in men's dress shoes. The good old American cowboy boot sports a pretty hefty heel in its own right, which probably helps those cowboys reach their horses better.

Many people think they don't wear high heels because they don't have on the "killers." Seems people are always trying to convince me that a heel doesn't really "count" if it's only an inch or two. Technically, however, a heel is considered "positive" when it is at *any* height above the rest of the foot. So while we tend to categorize high-heeled shoes based on how they look, from a health perspective *any* shoe with a positive heel is going to affect the geometry of the body.

Replacing the term "high heel" with "positive heel" will help you figure out which of your shoes are affecting how you move. When you start calling a spade a spade, you're going to notice that this new category of positive heel includes not only your traditional high heel but also the wedge, low pump…even your running shoe! Who knew?

Key Points, Chapter 5

1. Footwear can be complicated, but simply knowing more about the four key design areas can significantly impact the health of your feet.

2. The four areas to evaluate are the sole, the upper, the toe box, and the heel.

3. Each of these areas has the potential to limit the natural range of motion of the foot and toes.

4. From an engineering perspective, the heel of a shoe is considered positive when it is any height above the toes, meaning if you were to remove all the positive-heeled footwear from your closet—you might not have any shoes left!

CHAPTER 6

Shoe Science

"Think of the magic of that foot, comparatively small, upon which your whole weight rests. It's a miracle, and the dance ... is a celebration of that miracle."
—Martha Washington

Here is something you already know: your footwear can absolutely affect the performance of your outfit. But here is something you might not have known: your footwear can absolutely affect the performance of your body. You may wonder why geometry is important when talking about health. You may have been told that you wouldn't ever need to do math again, but guess what? The long-term function of your body depends on the way the particular bones, joints, and muscles are angled. Angled. There's a term from the math days long past. Before going on to how footwear characteristics affect your body position, let's talk about why geometry matters.

MUSCLES—THE LONG AND THE SHORT OF IT

The muscles in your body, after receiving an electrical signal from your brain, change from long to short. This change is called contraction, and it pulls on the bones of the body, which results in both the movement you see with your eyes, and the much smaller movements of fluids within the tissues. This smaller motion of fluid is called circulation, and the health of your entire body really depends on this process. Tissues that move frequently have better circulation than tissues that don't. The longer tissues go without circulation, the harder time they have continuing to grow (regenerate) at the correct rate.

So, back to geometry. Almost all of your muscles attach to bones. When you change the position of the bones, or limit the ability of the bones to arrange themselves into a particular configuration, you also affect the muscles that attach to those bones. The ability for a muscle to contract (which is how you get that circulation happening) depends on the length of the muscle. The shorter a muscle, the less it is able to change from one position to another. If a muscle is perpetually tight, it doesn't go through a full change, from long to short, which means it never circulates the full amount. The same process holds true for a muscle that is too long. Muscle tissue in either of these situations, being too long or too short, cannot generate the greatest amount of flow.

CIRCULATION—WHOSE JOB IS IT?

When we think of our blood circulating, we typically think of our heart as being the main driving force of blood throughout the body. In actuality, the same muscles that move your bones—your skeletal muscles—also play a significant role in getting the nutrient-rich blood distributed. The feet, being the farthest away from the heart, run the greatest risk of poor circulation. Blood is thick, and it is very hard to move when the muscles in the feet and lower leg are not doing much contracting to help out!

There are lots of factors that influence the movement of blood to the tissues, but if your feet have been locked up for a lifetime, training your foot muscles gives you a simple way that you can improve tissue health right now! See intrinsic foot strengtheners, pages 109–116.

Once you understand that skeletal position affects how the body works, it is much easier to understand why certain parts of your body aren't thriving. When it comes to ailments of the feet, it is also pretty easy to see how shoes can push the bones around, creating a physiological effect that most of us don't really think about. Muscles in the feet would do better at staying at the correct length if we were not constantly affecting the foot bones with our shoes. By limiting the ability for the foot bones to displace, we are minimizing the activity in the foot muscles. This limit in foot muscle activity means limited circulation in the feet. Limited circulation is bad news for the nerves, muscle, and skin of the feet and lower legs!

Shoes, in general, have characteristics that limit biological function, from reducing dynamic sensory input to limiting the ability for the foot to move relative to itself. It is the four anatomical parts of footwear, as described in Chapter 5, that are really the main culprits when it comes to affecting your whole-body geometry. Let's take a look at how each of the main shoe parts changes various joint angles.

THE SOLE

Before looking at what the sole of a shoe does, let us contemplate what the sole of a foot should be doing. In pre-footwear days, the sole of the foot both sensed the natural surfaces we once walked over and formed itself with each step to meet and maneuver over these surfaces. In order to comfortably adapt to changing surfaces, it is important to keep each of the foot's thirty-three joints and the numerous muscles as mobile as possible. This mobility also promotes the greatest amount of circulation to the tissue in the lower leg, giving us strong muscles, bones, and skin in the foot and the lower leg.

Just like your eyes and ears take in information about your environment, the skin is also a sense organ, and takes in information about qualities of the surfaces it contacts. Exposing the skin to varying surfaces creates a strong information highway between the feet and the brain, and the nerves conducting that highway are kept active and healthy.

NERVES OF THE FEET

There are two different types of nerves in the feet—motor nerves, which control the movement of the foot, and sensory nerves, which are responsible for "sensing" environmental factors like surface qualities (e.g., Am I stepping on something rough or smooth? Hot or cold?). Having both of these systems working optimally means that, in addition to every muscle in your feet being able to respond to the movement commands coming from the brain (have you mastered lifting your toes individually yet?), your feet are simultaneously "reading" the environment. This environmental information helps the user of the feet (that's you!) make rapid adjustments with the motor nerves, selecting where they step, and finding safe passages for the feet.

As I mentioned before, when shoes first appeared on the scene they were simple animal hides, tied to the soles with natural fibers. These soles were thin enough to maintain foot mobility, but thick enough to minimize risk of foot puncture. When foot puncture is a high risk, it obviously makes sense to pick a shoe that offers the greatest amount of safety—in the short term. The long-term use of this shoe, however, will decrease your foot sensitivity by limiting foot range of motion. This creates a deficiency in foot circulation as well as sensitivity, increasing your risk of a foot ailment. What a conundrum!

If that's not enough, there is one more risk to consider. Whenever a part of the body is unable to perform its job, other parts of the body will compensate. In the case of foot musculature that is impaired or unused, the ankle typically will develop compensatory movements, putting extra burden on that joint.

The moral to the sole: the thicker and stiffer the sole, the less the intrinsic foot musculature is able to do, the less communication happens between the brain and the feet, and the more compensatory movement at the ankle is increased.

THE UPPER

The upper portion of the shoe, when fitting correctly, would seem to limit foot function the least, right? After all, how much could a flimsy little flip-flop strap affect the gait pattern of a fully grown adult? Consider, for a moment, how a shoe stays on your foot. The upper is essentially a connection tool, designed to fasten the bottom of the shoe to your foot. As the upper gets smaller, so does the connection, saddling your foot with the responsibility of holding the shoe on.

Flip-flops, mules, and slide-on sandals are good examples of shoes that require a gripping action from the toes in order to keep the shoes from flying off while walking. This gripping motion of the toes is the same muscle pattern that deforms toe joints into the "hammertoe" position when done over and over again. If you don't believe me, try walking in these shoes keeping your toes relaxed. It's fairly impossible! This gripping reflex is so strong it happens automatically, which means that if you have hammertoes, and you are wearing a shoe with a minimal upper, you are training your toes into the gripping motion with each step. That's not what you were intending to do, was it?

THE TOE BOX

The muscles of the toes tend to get away with doing very little over our modern lifetimes, as they have been squished into toe boxes since our first years. Throughout history, the square footprint has often been considered to be less attractive culturally, creating societal norms that include foot binding, and the more subtle (but equally unnatural) tight toe boxes found throughout fashion today.

Just like a plaster cast limits the motion of a joint, resulting in muscle atrophy, the narrow toe space of most footwear prevents the spreading of the toes away from each other. Chronic toe squeezing not only weakens the muscles of the toes but also loads the bones while they are positioned incorrectly, increasing the occurrence of joint stress, bone stress, and other soft tissue deformation. Ouch!

Because the square footprint was considered to be more "native" and therefore less desirable by the upper classes, it is no wonder the small foot aesthetic has been passed down from generation to generation. Out of all of the footwear characteristics, the squeezing of the toes into tight boxes has no functional or safety purpose; it is just a design component that has been elevated to the preferred look. A toe box that provides enough space for toe spreading, however, allows the toes and their joints to load in their correct positions, decreasing unnecessary stress.

ABDUCTION AND ADDUCTION

The terms abduction and adduction are anatomical terms that are used to describe what a motion looks like. Abduction means "to move away from a midline." When the toes abduct, you can see them spread away from each other, creating space between the toes.

Adduction means the opposite. Just like "add" means to bring two numbers together, adduction means "to bring toward the midline." Adduction is the muscular action that brings the toes toward each other. Shoes (especially tight toe boxes) often keep the toes adducted. When your toes are adducted, there is no space between them.

Practice abducting and adducting your toes, trying to limit the curling or gripping action. Ideally, the toes can open and close as easily as you abduct and adduct your fingers!

THE HEEL

There are a lot of parts to a shoe, but no footwear component is quite as detrimental—or as researched—as the positive heel. Why is everyone shocked that high heels are often linked to foot, knee, and back pain? Have you ever worn high heels? Have you ever *danced* in high heels?

When it comes to geometry, the positive heel creates an instant change in foot angle that cannot be eliminated as long as the shoe is on the foot. I always chuckle when people spend money on "proving" that the heel affects body position. It's geometry. It's the tenth-grade stuff that one could figure out in high school, if one just knew the basic principles!

We all start our rationalization at the same place: the small heel of a shoe hardly seems like enough to cause great problems. Keep in mind, however, that although the height of a short heel may just be one or two inches, the foot is relatively short in length compared to the height of the body, so the number of degrees that a one- or two-inch heel can displace you is quite large. What other machine do you know that you expect long-term use from in positions that are twenty, thirty, or forty degrees off their normal axis? Would you want to drive your car with the wheels twenty to forty degrees out of alignment? What if your washing machine was perched at a forty-degree angle?

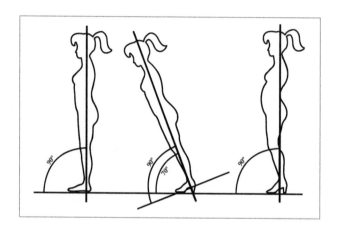

The higher the heel, the greater you move your good alignment (the first figure) into the compensating posture (the third figure). The middle figure demonstrates the amount of malalignment you have to deal with coming from your heel. A person can compensate for the high, forward pitch with their ankles, knees, pelvic tilt, or spinal curvature. Any one of these joints can be displaced to make the heel wearer look fairly upright, even if their bones are not truly vertical or loaded optimally.

The *way* a person compensates for their heel is based on many factors—their postural preferences and habits, the lengths of their body segments, their gait, and injury history. That is what makes it difficult to generalize the precise negative effects that raised heels create; each person copes with her displacement differently. But even if the compensations vary, the angular displacement is precise, and is fairly easy to calculate if you do a simple calculation of heel height and foot-segment length.

In addition to whole-body displacement, the positive heel also instantly increases the load on the front of the foot. Decreasing this load is very important, especially for those with forefoot ailments and toe issues. Just reducing the heel on a shoe will instantly decrease the loading that is increasing the pressure and furthering the issue.

"FIT SHOES"

A whole new category of shoes has recently come onto the market—"fit shoes." Distinct from athletic shoes, these are shoes whose makers claim, explicitly or implicitly, that you will become more fit simply by wearing them. Because these shoes have various features that are unique to their brands, they can affect your mechanics differently.

At the writing of this book, the feature that fitness shoe designers were fiddling with most in order to affect the body was the sole. Decreasing the sole stability seems to be a common theme in fit footwear, with the theory that if a surface is unstable, the body will have to use more muscle in order to stabilize itself. That absolutely makes sense from a physical training perspective. The result of using new muscle is usually an increase in overall fitness level, for as muscle mass develops so do things like total body lean mass and resting metabolism rate.

However, not all muscle development is good for the body's structural longevity. For example, an exercise like the shoulder shrug can develop the muscles that lift the shoulders up toward the ears. Great! Now I have firm traps and more muscle mass. The tension that develops in this muscle, though, decreases the amount of space for the spinal disks in my neck. Not so great. So while it is easy to think that any muscle development is good, there are many, many cases where it is not. The arbitrary development of muscle, while perhaps contributing to overall muscle mass, may have negative effects on the health of a joint or tendon.

The best way to evaluate your favorite fit shoe brand is to see how it holds up against our four-factor evaluation:

THE SOLE: Does the sole allow natural movement of the foot, or does it make the bulk of motion come from the ankle?

THE UPPER: Do I have to grip my toes to keep this shoe on, or does it connect well?

THE TOE BOX: Can my toes spread comfortably, or is spreading space reduced by a too-narrow toe box?

THE HEEL: Is the heel on this shoe affecting my other joints, or can I maintain a truly vertical alignment?

FAST FOOT MATH

For those math nerds out there, the foot presents a fascinating math problem, just waiting to be solved. If I asked you how many unique positions you could achieve with your fingers, it would seem to be an infinite amount—in fact, just playing one song on the piano would exercise your fingertips beyond their comfort zone.

There is a mathematical way, however, to solve problems like these. When trying to find out all of the possible ways your foot can be deformed, you only need to apply a mathematical term called a factorial. Factorials are used to figure out the number of unique ways different variables can be organized. In a foot with thirty-three joints, using a factorial means we multiply thirty-three times thirty-two times thirty-one times thirty...all the way down to one. There is a button on most calculators that will do this for you that has an exclamation point as its symbol.

Thirty-three factorial (33! in calculator-speak) comes out to equal 8.68 x 1036 different ways your foot can be deformed (or 8,600,000,000,000,000, 000,000,000,000,000,000,000). This unfathomably high number shows the potential of the nerves and muscles of our feet if we challenged them over a lifetime.

INSPECT YOUR FOOTWEAR

Aided by your new knowledge of footwear, you can now cast a more objective eye on the pair of shoes you wear the most often.

FOUR-FACTOR EVALUATION

If wearing shoes...	Best	Not too bad	Hard on the body	
Heel	Negative or flat	Minimal positive	Positive, 1-2"	Positive, more than 2"
Toe Box	Toes move freely	Toes have some space	Toes can't move	Toes are squished
Upper	Well-attached	Sandal with heel strap	Slide	Flip-flop
Sole	Thin and flexible	Flexible, even if not so thin	Rigid, even if not so thick	Thick and rigid

CINDERELLA, DOES THE SHOE FIT?

Most women have spent their entire lives wearing shoes that are too small. Because we've been wearing them this way for so long, the sensation of tightly held feet seems quite normal. In fact, to many folks, shoes feel sloppy when they aren't pressing into the tissues of the feet. To get a sense of how much your shoes are affecting your foot mechanics, let's see how your shoes measure up against your feet, literally.

Try this: while standing, step onto a piece of paper without shoes or socks, and trace all around the outside of your foot (if you have a child to help you, they love this task!).

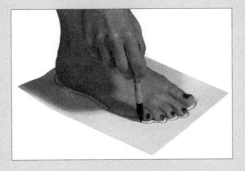

Step off and take a look at the size of your foot drawing. This is the true shape your foot should be allowed to take while under the load of your body weight.

CONTINUED ON NEXT PAGE...

Now, take out a few pairs of your favorite shoes and see how their size compares to the tracing. Many times, people will find their footwear is much narrower, especially at the toe box, than their foot actually is wide.

Key Points, Chapter 6

1. Muscle plays a role in circulation, which is necessary to keep tissues healthy.
2. The position of the skeleton affects how much muscle can contract, which, in turn, affects the quantity of circulation coming through a particular area.
3. Footwear characteristics can instantly impact the position of your bones or the angle of your joints.
4. By knowing which footwear component affects each aspect of foot health, you can make better choices to improve your particular ailments.

CHAPTER 7

Women...Undermining Women's Health

"Sacrifice for beauty."
—MY GRANDMOTHER

A ll over the "civilized" world, women are suffering from physical ailments that they may or may not understand. Have women been granted less-than-adequate physical bodies? Are our feet prone to chronic pain due to some hormonal issue? Are we just so weak, brittle, and fragile that daily life is causing our bodies to spontaneously break down? Is it these ailments that have granted us the distinction of the weaker sex, or is there something more logical and more mechanical going on?

When it comes to the feet, the statistics point to a higher incidence of pain in women. They also show a correlation between certain footwear characteristics and functional limitations in these women as they age. In an age of scientific research, one would assume that the reason this particular pitfall of women's health continues would be a lack of clinical data. But this is not so. There is enough research on footwear and inappropriate joint movements, excessive pressure, increased loading, increased risk of hip fractures, links to knee osteoarthritis, and alterations in pelvic placement and spinal curvature for someone in charge to say, "Your shoes, ma'am, might be making you sick."

It is easy to blame the current state of women's health on a historical lack of research, or a previous apathy toward women's issues in general. Feeling like a victim to our current physical pain or ailments is also an easy path. When taking a closer look at the link between our habits, our personal choices, and the constant struggle between what we know is the "right" thing to do health-wise and what we tend to do, choosing poorly is an age-old habit.

Now granted, to a certain degree you may have already known this. Somewhere, your good judgment must have had a reaction to a particular pair of shoes—you know, the ones you can't walk in for longer than an hour. Let's say that you only had an inkling in your subconscious. But let us say, now, that you know better. You know better, but you still want to wear things that make you feel pretty and confident. I get it—totally. I've read Cinderella, too—Big Feet=Ugly Spinster Stepsisters. Ugly spinster stepsisters still living at home. To win the prince's heart, and live happily ever after, you must cram your foot into this tiny glass slipper. Seriously. Run that glass slipper through the four footwear evaluation points and you will find that while the upper passes the test, the heel is too high, the toe box is big enough for only two toes, and the sole flexibility is zero. Good luck with that.

> *My first pair of high heels were the plastic ones they used to, and maybe still do, sell in the "girl" kits you'd find in the drugstore toy section. They often came with gaudy clip-on earrings, lip gloss, and such. I was about seven years old and wore them to bed the first couple of nights. That phase died out in me pretty quickly, thankfully, since I was one of the taller girls in school, not to mention a creature of comfort. Those darn things hurt! These days I prefer to be barefoot... which makes me truly feel like a little girl again.*
>
> —AMBER N.

Women love shoes. It's a fact. I am not sure if it is a re-searched fact, but I can confidently call it anecdotal. Women also get more from their shoes than simply covering the foot. Footwear changes the way we feel about ourselves. Shoes can make you feel taller if you're petite, or authoritative when you need to gather power. Shoes change the visual propor-tions of an outfit, distorting (subjectively improving) the way your body looks to others. And...shoes always fit, even when the clothes don't. Shoes are important because shoes make us feel better *psychologically*. And that is great, right up until they make us actually worse *physically*.

Early in 2010, a study came out about the harmful ef-fects of heels and was covered on a national news show. The female anchor interviewing a doctor about what the study meant stated clearly, on national television, that it did not matter how bad they were for her, she would not be giving her heels up—ever. I couldn't help but think that this attitude, of knowingly doing harm to one's own body, is, let's face it, really stupid. The science is there. The research is there. The pain is there. The visits to the doctor are there. Are we really feeling so badly about who we are that we have to pay for fashion with our health?

There have been other products in our culture that have provided the same psychological benefits—making us feel sexier, thinner, and more sophisticated—even though, simultaneously, they were wreaking negative effects on our physiology.

THE NO HIGH-HEEL SECTION

As a regular blogger, I came across a nutritional website asking if fast food would become the cigarettes of the future. I disagreed with the notion. There aren't many doctors across America who are going to be eating out of a greasy sack while you are sitting across the desk getting a prescription for high-blood pressure medication. I posted my own comment, arguing that the positive-heeled shoe would eventually be found to be the main instigator in expensive ailments of not only the feet but of the knees, hips, and spine as well.

My post was:

> I don't think fast food has become the "new smoking" as much as high heels have. Once upon a time, the

rationale for smoking was the sex appeal and the positive effect on weight management. Because it is hard to rationalize the choice of donuts as a positive one, poor food choices don't fit as smoothly into the analogy.

Bone density-decreasing, nerve-damaging, and arthritis-causing high heels are probably being worn by your favorite OBGYN during your annual exam, eerily reminiscent of a 1950s doctor's visit, where Mr. Doctor chain smoked throughout your entire exam (anyone out there watch Mad Men?*).*

Blind to the detrimental effects footwear has on health, or the correlation of footwear to the gait alterations happening in the mother-to-be waiting in her office, Ms. High-Heel-Wearing Women's Health Specialist doesn't know, in the exact same way Mr. Smoking MD didn't know, that when you look at the heeled shoe, you are looking at the "cigarettes" of the future.

I know, I know. Likening shoes to cigarettes is a pretty bold statement. And calling out doctors in heels as promoting poor health is also fairly bold. But think of this: a long, long time ago the cigarette, an item most would agree has a huge, negative impact on your health, was promoted by health care workers because there was no literature or research stating clearly that smoking was harmful to your health—until there was. And then there was a long time where people disagreed about what the research meant. And then it took a lot of time before people who smoked were able to stop, including people who truly understood the negative effects. Finally, smoking ended up on the list of clearly marked risk factors for many ailments, and insurance companies started taking note of who smoked and who didn't before giving people coverage. And if my prediction is right, so it will go with positive-heeled footwear.

INTRINSIC VERSUS EXTRINSIC MOTIVATORS

We have all decided to start a program at some point in time, whether for exercise or otherwise. What makes us successful at staying with these programs lies in what motivated us to start them.

Extrinsic motivating factors for exercise programs come from outside, like your doctor suggesting you begin a movement program for weight loss, or receiving a reward for completing a task.

Intrinsic motivation comes from the doer, as a result of the sheer pleasure or benefit one gets from the task.

Although you may have begun your foot health program in response to nagging pain (an extrinsic factor) or at someone else's suggestion, understanding the benefits and feeling good after finishing each exercise can shift your motivation to intrinsic. Intrinsic motivation has been found to be an essential component of long-term success when it comes to physical improvement!

Until the research—research that already exists—begins to register on the radar screens of the people in charge of distributing health information to the public, there are things you can do to stop the perpetuation of the prevailing female footwear paradigm. Just say "No!" to harmful shoes and "Yes!" to beautiful shoes that not only complement you and your outfit but also the long-term function of your human machine.

Realize that whatever look you are trying to achieve in killer footwear while standing in front of a mirror, people are looking at the whole package, which includes how you move. Nothing says "youthful" like a smooth, symmetrical gait. Nothing says, "Hi, I am old and injured, so if you are a lion feel free to pick me off from the herd" like a gimpy limp. Work on your gait ASAP!

If you are a health care professional, understand that by modeling your own poor footwear choices, you are endorsing them as acceptable. You wouldn't smoke during an examination, would you? Both lung and joint tissue should have the chance to function optimally. And whether or not you feel it is your job description, you are a role model for health and wellness.

If you have or work with children, teach them that footwear cannot possibly give them the self-esteem that should be coming from within. Shoes—just like smoking—may make them feel cool, but in the end they can increase physical suffering.

I have to admit, when I first learned about high heels and the damage they cause, I was sure I could "cut back" and wear flats more often. But after a year of learning more and more about alignment, and buying my first pair of negative-heeled shoes, I find that now I hardly ever wear anything but flats. In fact, even my favorite cowboy boots, with their two-inch heel, are gathering dust in my closet. Now that my feet don't hurt, and my toes are spread, there is no way I would stuff them all into a pointy-toed high heel. Plus, I feel more GROUNDED, better balanced, and am always ready for a long walk. THANK YOU for speaking out on this subject.

—VICKI A.

A little reminder: there is adequate research stating the harmful effects of footwear on the health of the human body. Even though the masses may not be dealing with this issue right now, you can still benefit from the diligent work done by many researchers, knowing that you can take control over your own level of health.

WHY IS REPAIRING YOUR FEET SUCH A BIG DEAL?

The function of the foot goes way beyond the scrunching of the toes and the stabilizing of the ankle. The foot is the platform for your entire body. The muscles have to be strong enough to keep your entire body moving as smoothly as possible. If I haven't clearly stated it before, the current state of your feet is a future projection of how well you will be able to move as you get older.

If you are already having problems with your feet, the problem is bigger than just the current nagging issue. Even though this book primarily addresses your feet, the health of a lot of other tissue in the body depends on the state of their health. You may have never really thought about it before, but consider this: your ability to walk and balance depends on the mobility and the strength of the muscles within the foot. This is important because your ability to maintain a level of function simpatico with independent living requires that you both walk and balance to a degree that it is safe to do so.

Okay, enough with the scare tactics. Let's say you aren't worried about future living arrangements. How about foot pain limiting the ability to maintain your weight? If you have foot pain, you more than likely are not going to start that necessary whole-body movement program. Walking, the most beneficial exercise you can do for your cardiovascular system, depends on the health of your feet! If they are too sore to go out, then none of you gets to go.

You'd have to be living under a rock that's under a giant heap of dirt that's under another larger rock to have missed the fact that a healthy body needs regular movement. Millions of people schlep themselves to the gym or yoga class, or head outside for a walk, to check off this daily to-do on the health list, and that's great. But what most people don't know is, they have unwittingly neglected the large portion of muscles that live below the ankle. Often the most "fit" individuals—athletes, dancers, aerobics instructors, and marathon runners—have the least healthy feet. This painful truth is often blamed on overuse of the feet instead of where it actually belongs—on the physiological cause of pounding the tissues of the feet into the ground without appropriate muscle training, and the habit of wearing tissue-weakening footwear.

Whatever your motivation is at this point—whether it's a reduction in foot pain, preventive medicine, interest in restoring alignment, or just plain curiosity—you are now armed with enough information to move into the exercise portion of this book!

Key Points, Chapter 7

1. Women often use footwear for "feel-good" reasons, which can make footwear habits hard to give up.
2. High heels may someday be looked at the same way that we now look at cigarettes, which also were once thought of as highly fashionable.
3. There is an abundance of published research showing that footwear is a contributing factor to musculoskeletal ailments of the foot, knees, hip, and spine. Because of the limits on how information is spread, this knowledge has not yet become widely known.
4. You do not have to wait for this information to become generally accepted knowledge before you can improve your situation—you can start using research findings now.

5. Foot health affects other tissue beyond your feet, making it essential to begin your foot-health program as soon as you can!

CHAPTER 8

The Foot Gym

"The first step towards getting somewhere is to decide that you are not going to stay where you are."
—John Pierpont Morgan

No matter the state of your feet (or your shoe closet!) you can absolutely make significant progress on your foot health with a little exercise intervention and habit modification. The great thing about human tissue is that it adapts easily, at any age. Really—it does. Before getting started with this exercise program, take a few moments to figure out which level of foot training you should start with.

Which statement best fits you?

STATEMENT ONE

1. I regularly go barefoot.

2. I wear high-heeled shoes to work often, but also wear flats or pad around my house in bare feet.
3. My feet are so sore, my doctor has recommended wearing shoes all the time.

STATEMENT TWO

1. I've never really worn high heels except for a few dressy occasions.
2. I have about four to five pairs of positive-heeled shoes (one to two inches) in my closet that I wear regularly.
3. I wore high heels today to work. In fact, I'm wearing them right now, as I read this book curled up on the couch.

STATEMENT THREE

1. I jog or run regularly, usually four to five times per week.
2. I walk at least three times a week, and do some light stretching.
3. Balance has gotten more difficult for me. I don't feel comfortable standing on one foot without something to hold on to.

If you answered mostly Threes, it is likely the tissue in your feet is extremely stiff. You will be starting with stretches of shorter duration and can use a chair or wall for extra balance as needed.

If you answered mostly Twos, you should be able to shoot for the midrange of exercise time. You may find that doing the exercise more often, with a lower holding time, will be your best bet.

If you answered mostly Ones, then your feet, while still in need of specific strengthening, are probably up for the full recommended sixty-second holds for each exercise. Some exercises may be more challenging than others, especially for athletes who have overused but undertrained their feet.

Because most of us have been wearing shoes since an early age, we have missed out on learning the motions and exercising 25 percent of our muscles. The exercises in the "Foot Gym" affect the little muscles of the toes and those that support the arch of the foot, and also include the larger muscles down the back and sides of the thigh. These exercises are designed to not only undo years of accumulated damage in the feet and ankles but will also help align the hip joints to increase bone density and position the pelvic floor muscles for better bladder control and organ support.

PREPARING SPACE TO TRAIN YOUR FEET

To truly repair the foot, exercises for the feet need to be done without shoes. For those who have advanced neuropathy or diabetes, a concern is stepping on items that can puncture your foot without you feeling it. If you have very stiff feet, exercising on hard surfaces can also be challenging. To keep your feet safe, prepare a barefoot-friendly space before doing your exercises.

- Run a vacuum over your exercise space. A good vacuum will pick up smaller, hard-to-see items like sewing needles, pins, and tacks.
- Clear enough space to roll out a yoga mat or a large bath towel. This will give you an extra protective layer.
- For extra-sensitive feet, place your exercise mat on carpet, or layer a blanket or multiple towels to cushion your exercise space.
- Do a final, visual check for any potentially missed items.

These exercises require attention to detail. There are many things that change the effectiveness of an exercise, like the position of the feet, the bend in the knees, and the pitch of the torso. Learning where your entire body should be while stretching will help you target the exact muscle fibers you are intending to lengthen, and increase the overall effectiveness of the program.

Exercise One: Stretching the Calves

The muscles in the calves are considered part of the extrinsic foot muscle group, but when it comes to the long-term effects of the positive heel, the back of the leg is significantly impacted. Long-term positive-heel wearing has been shown to shorten the fibers in the lower leg by 13 percent. Thirteen percent!

I know that you may think you already stretch your calves, but that's because you have never met *this* calf stretch before. There are many different versions of a calf stretch, and most have been given some type of stretch for this part of the body at some time or another, but not all calf stretches are created equal!

For this exercise, you will need:

- A full-size bathroom towel, folded and rolled
- A chair or a wall for balance

Start standing, facing the rolled towel.

Place the ball of one foot on the rolled towel, and gently lower your heel to the floor. Take a few seconds to straighten both legs all the way, keeping the thigh muscles relaxed. Once you've gotten used to this position, take a small step forward with the other leg.

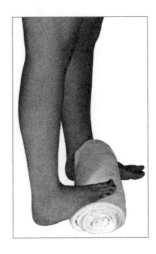

If your body starts leaning forward, or you have to bend either knee, scoot the foot on the floor back until you can maintain the stretch. Use a wall or chair for balance if you feel wobbly. Step back and repeat on the other side.

ATTENTION PELVIC THRUSTERS

Once you have taken a few passes at the calf stretch, start paying attention to the placement of the hips. The weight of the pelvis should stay directly over the stretching leg. Back your hips up until they stack vertically over the ankle and knee of the back leg. Maintain this hip position as you try to stretch your opposite foot further forward.

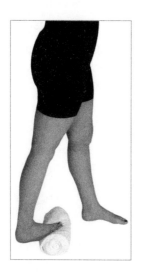 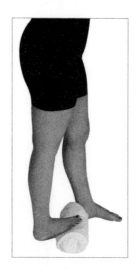

Wrong way (left): the pelvis moves forward of the back ankle.
Right way (right): the pelvis stays stacked over the back ankle.

OTHER POSTURES TO WATCH

If your torso is leaning forward while stretching your legs, you have stepped too far forward. Shorten your "stride" until your body is stacked vertically. Only increase the distance between the feet if you can maintain your upright posture!

Helpful Tips: The thickness of the rolled towel makes this stretch more or less intense. If your ankle feels stiff, use a thinner towel, or don't roll it up all the way. If stretching on this lower surface is still too intense, back the foot up just a bit to decrease the angle in the ankle. The same holds true for making the stretch more intense. For a greater stretch, choose a thicker or longer towel!

Why is this stretch so important?

Optimal, upright walking should be an act that does little to damage the tissues. People, however, have developed a "falling instead of walking" habit that causes excessive loads on the joints and bones. The correct length of the calf muscle would allow a step to happen without extreme pulling down the back of the leg, which will shorten your stride in the long run.

The calf stretch is an easy way to measure how far you can step without being "jerked back" by the calf. This stretch is also a great way to regain some of the muscle length stolen from years of positive-heeled shoes. The longer you have worn heels, and the higher those heels are, the more challenging this stretch will be. Be patient and gentle with this stretch. If you have had a lifetime of muscle shortening in the lower leg, you can't undo it in thirty days. What you can do to increase the length is slowly wean yourself down to a lower heel and then to a flat, as well as pay attention to where your hips and torso are while walking around. Keep yourself vertical!

Exercise Two: Stretching the "Gripping" Muscles

Although I am a fan of movement for health, not every exercise is beneficial for every person at each stage of her life. Instead, some can actually worsen conditions because of the way they cause the muscles to shorten, and how that shortening affects the joints involved. "Towel scrunching" or "marble lifting" is a common foot-strengthening exercise often recommended to patients with weak or stiff feet, hoping that the increase in movement will help fix the issue. While this towel scrunching could possibly benefit someone with general foot or ankle weakness stemming from recent surgery, I am not a fan of this particular exercise as a long-term, beneficial, mechanical habit.

Just like the mechanics of wearing flip-flops, this toe-gripping action promotes a further shortening of the muscles in the toes that can lead to a decrease in joint range of motion. This "toe scrunching" motion is also the very same muscle pattern that can lead to hammertoes!

Tight forefoot muscles stemming from overloading the front of the foot as a result of positive heels, excessive flip-flop wearing, or just years of poor posture can generate tight, gripping toes.

This exercise not only stretches out the front of the ankle but also the toes if they have the gripping habit!

For this exercise you will need:

- A chair and/or wall to aid in balance

There are two ways to begin this exercise. If you are a Three in terms of exercise readiness (see pages 93–94), then start seated. Ones and Twos can start standing, unless you prefer otherwise.

Reach one foot behind you, allowing the tops of the toes to touch the floor. If you are standing, you can start by reaching back from the knee, or, to make the stretch more challenging, you can reach back from the hip. Try to keep both knees straight and your body upright. Be aware of your pelvis—it will tend to thrust forward to minimize the stretch!

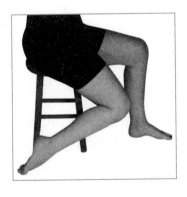 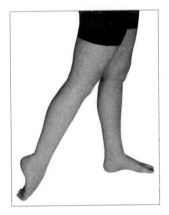

ATTENTION TO DETAIL

When the feet are very tight, the ankle will tend to roll out to the side (incorrect), overloading the outer toes. Bring the ankle back toward your midline (correct), keeping the weight evenly distributed over the big and smaller toes!

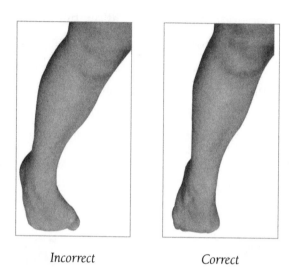

Incorrect   *Correct*

Note: Cramping in the toes is very common while stretching them out after years of tensing them with every step. Feel free to start stretching in short bursts of time, seconds even, going back from foot to foot. You will notice the cramping subsides with regular practice.

WHEN WILL MY "GRIPPERS" RELAX?

If getting your toes to release is your main priority, take a look at your footwear of choice. If you regularly wear shoes with minimal uppers, shoes like flip-flops, poorly connecting sandals, mules, or clogs, your hammertoe muscles are working overtime to keep your shoes on. And all the muscle length you acquire via exercise will be gone as soon as you tense your feet again.

If you have discovered you like to wear your pelvis out in front of you, or are fond of the positive heel, you might be causing the muscles to tense under the extra forefoot load. Reducing your heel over time, getting yourself back down to the ground, and minding your pelvis will help you keep your toe muscles relaxed and increase the long-term effectiveness of all of your foot exercises!

Exercise Three: Lengthen the Backs of the Legs

When you have worn positive heels (and who hasn't worn positive-heeled shoes) over a lifetime, the tension can affect not only the muscles in the lower leg but also the connective tissues running down the back of the thigh. Super-tight calf muscles can become super-tight hamstrings, especially if you have adapted to the geometrical changes of your shoes by slightly bending the knees. To move this stretch up a bit higher, we will add another piece of the puzzle.

For this exercise you will need:

- A chair
- A rolled towel

Start standing with straight feet, facing the seat of a chair. Bend forward, letting the hands settle flat against the seat of a chair. Back your pelvis up, until your hips are slightly behind your ankles. You may need to step a bit closer to the chair to do this easily.

If the backs of your legs are very tight, your muscles will pull your tailbone down to the floor. In this position, try to gently lift your tailbone up, away from the floor, increasing the stretch down the back of the leg.

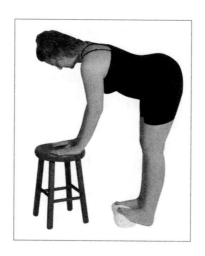

If your pelvis is extremely tucked in this exercise, stay at it with your feet flat on the ground. To increase the stretch, however, you can add the rolled towel under the front of the foot. Just like in the single-calf stretch, the height of the rolled towel affects the intensity of the stretch. For more stretch, increase the thickness of the towel; for less stretch, decrease the thickness, or remove the towel altogether.

SHOES DID ALL OF THIS?

I would like to point out that, as a culture, we have not been very kind to our posterior leg muscles. Not only has chronic footwear use tightened the back of the legs but excessive hours of sitting every day has also contributed to the shortening of these muscles. Stretching the backs of the legs can (and should) be done throughout the day, especially if you are a professional sitter. Keep a towel in a desk drawer at work for a quick leg lengthener three to four times a workday.

Exercise Four: Using the Wall

This is another, more relaxing way to stretch the back of the entire leg. Oftentimes, tight lower-leg muscles will cause the feet to point away from the up position while performing regular stretches. Using a wall prevents that movement from creeping in, and increases the effectiveness of this leg stretch.

For this exercise you will need:

- A pillow or sitting cushion
- A wall

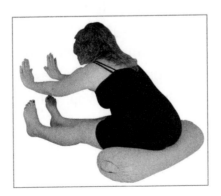

Begin by sitting with your legs stretched out in front of you. Sitting up on a rolled towel, pillow, or sitting cushion will help tight hamstrings and make this stretch a bit more comfortable. Scoot your body toward a wall, placing the soles of both feet flat against the wall. Pay special attention to your heels, making sure they are firmly pressed into the wall.

Relax your thighs. The knees should not be bent, nor should they be forced to the ground. If your legs are so tight that they cannot straighten all the way, you can back away from the wall, allowing your feet to relax slightly.

Slowly relax your body forward, trying to bend at the hips instead of the spine. If you can, reach your hands out to the wall. At this point, you can place your palms against the wall, or brush your fingertips against the wall or stare longingly at the wall. Find the option that works best for you. Finally, you can allow the neck to relax, letting the head drop forward. Take relaxing breaths and no bouncing.

WHY NO BOUNCING?

Bouncing while you stretch is called ballistic stretching. Often found in martial arts, the vigorous technique of a fast stretch and release has a place in sports where the body may need to prepare for the fast joint changes found in contact events. Unless you are planning on being attacked in the next few days, the muscle tissue really needs a long, steady pull to change tension habits. Adjust your behavior accordingly.

Exercises Five through 10: Toe Lifts

Remember those small muscles within the foot, the intrinsic muscles? Just like your fingers move individually, so should your toes. Because the toes have been tightly bound for perhaps all of your life, this exercise takes a while to master. In fact, toe lifts are actually five exercises rolled up into one!

For this exercise you will need:

- Your feet

Start with bare feet, pointing straight ahead. See if you can isolate the muscles that lift the big toe, getting it to lift off the ground, without taking any of the other toes with it!

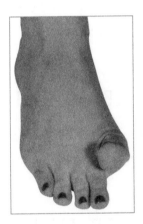

If this is easy, you can move on, following the big toe lift with a second, third, fourth, and finally, fifth toe.

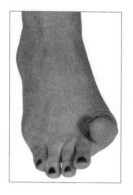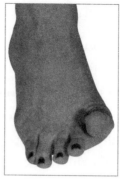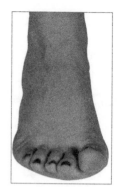

When lifting the toes individually, the foot and ankle should not change position, meaning you should not roll your ankle slightly to help you get the toes up. They have muscles of their own!

If you are having a hard time getting started, you can lean forward to hold the other toes down to help your brain isolate the tissue you are trying to use.

WANT ANOTHER CHALLENGE?

After you have developed the ability to lift your toes up, one at a time, you can also practice setting them back down in order.

WANT ANOTHER, EVEN MORE CHALLENGING CHALLENGE?

Once you have mastered lifting and lowering your toes in order, you can practice lifting each toe off the ground, by itself. This is much more challenging. Try picking up only your second toe. All of the other toes have to stay glued to the ground. Once you have figured out how to do that, you can start working on your third, fourth, and fifth toes. This one takes a long (long) time to master, so get to it!

GOT BUNIONS?

If you have developed *hallux valgus* along the way, pay attention to the big toe as it lifts off the ground. Does it come straight up, or does it also veer off toward the pinky toe when lifting? In addition to your lifting muscles, you can take this opportunity to begin the arduous task of strengthening the big toe abductor (the muscle that stretches the big toe away from the others) while doing your lifts. Who knew doing foot exercises could make you break a mental sweat?

Exercise 11: Toe Spreading

Toes that have been crammed into tight toe boxes adapt to the limited space by squeezing together. This causes the muscles that pull the toes together (the adductors) to become tight and stiff, and the muscles that pull the toes away from each other (the abductors) to become weak.

A simple exercise to strengthen the toe-spreading muscles is to do just that; spread them! As often as you can, whether while barefoot or even when trapped in shoes, think toe spread!

For this exercise you will need:

- A foot

- A hand
- Something to sit on

Start by looking down at your parallel bare feet. Try to move the toes away from each other, creating space between each toe. Can you see the floor between them? As you try to get them to move away from each other, notice if they tend to lift up off the floor or scrunch up in interesting patterns. This is all part of the process of learning a new movement program.

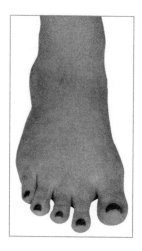

When you first start, the toes might not go very far. After all, it may have been thirty, forty, or even more than fifty years since you've played with your feet! To help them spread a bit more easily, try this stretch for the muscles in between the toes, or the toe's "inner thighs" as I like to call them.

HOLD HANDS WITH YOUR FEET

Sit in a comfortable position where you can get to your toes easily (crossing one leg over your knee works best). Place one fingertip between the tips of each toe, starting as far away from your foot as possible. Just placing your fingers in between your toes will give you a good stretch, but as these muscles begin to restore their length, you can work your fingers farther down, until eventually, your fingers "hold hands" with your feet.

For more toe stretching, you can slightly spread your fingers, which will, in turn, move the toes away from each other even more. You can choose how much you want to stretch your feet. Give yourself plenty of time (weeks, months, years) to improve your foot health. After all, it took a long time to get your feet to their current state!

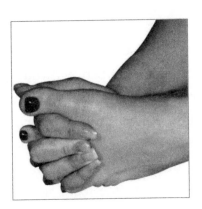

After taking your fingers out, try standing up and using your spreading muscles on their own. Are you able to spread better now?

Note: If you cannot get to your toes easily, you can ask someone for help. A massage therapist can help you with this stretch—or, you can usually pay one of your kids a dollar (or five) to do it for you.

HOW LONG UNTIL MY TOES SPREAD EASILY?

Keep in mind that most shoes squish your toes together every minute that you wear them, so to undo hours of damage, hours of stretch are needed. Don't worry—I don't expect you to sit around with your fingers between your toes that entire time. There are a few inexpensive solutions that can work on your feet *for* you, while you are reading, watching television, or even sleeping.

If you've ever had a professional pedicure, you have probably had soft foam padding placed between each of your toes. These "toe spacers" can be found at most beauty supply or drug stores and are usually less than five dollars. Pick up a pair and try popping them between your toes and let them stretch your toes while you sit back and relax. Or relax as much as you can, while your toes are ripped away from each other. Just kidding. Stretching just feels like that sometimes, especially when you've been hard on your feet!

The one drawback to the foam spacers is they tend to stretch out after a few uses and are difficult to walk around or sleep in. Thankfully, there are new products on the market that are designed for this exact purpose. My favorite "spreading" invention is the newer toe-alignment socks because you can walk around in them without your spacers falling out, they are softer than other spreading devices, and you can wash them in the machine.

> *Our mother put us in sensible brown oxfords all through grade school and we hated her for it! When we reached the ripe old age of eleven, we were allowed to pick out and wear whatever shoe types we wanted. I was in love with a pair of light blue flats, which I bought in a size 7 1/2 even though my foot measured a size 8 1/2!!!!! I paid a dear price for trying to have my feet appear smaller! Years later, I have bunions, hammertoes, fallen arches, and one very bad arthritic knee!*
>
> *Thank you, Katy, for introducing me to proper foot alignment and better shoes so that at sixty-four years of age, I'm finally able to spread my toes, have decreased the angle of my bunions and height of my hammertoes, and can now walk for at least an hour with no knee pain!!!!*
>
> —CHRIS D.

Exercise 12: Get On the Ball

The foot was designed to walk long distances over natural surfaces. These surfaces were not only bumpy and rocky paths but also yielding sands and firmly packed dirt. Natural ground also includes various and random changes in surface. The contours of the earth kept our feet supple by requiring them to form around many different objects. After wearing shoes for our entire lives, stepping on objects feels excruciating, even smooth and broad stones that in no way pose a threat to puncturing our princess feet!

Because the foot is often held against a flat, unchanging surface in the shoe, the numerous joints in the foot are not encouraged to move individually. Stepping on surfaces that vary in size and shape is what keeps joints mobile, so to innervate, or "wake up" these areas, you're going to get on the ball!

For largely immobile feet, starting with a tennis ball is a safe way to introduce joint movement you have, more than likely, never experienced.

For this exercise, you will need:

- A tennis ball

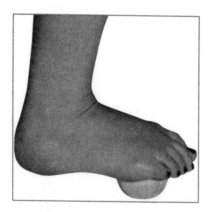

Start by placing just the front of the foot on the ball. Let your foot drape gently over the ball. When you are working with the ball, always keep your heel down on the ground. Keep both of your feet side by side and slowly move your foot forward, one inch at a time, spending twenty to thirty seconds "just standing" with the ball underneath that area. Once you have worked as far back as you can without lifting your heel, switch to the other foot.

Once you have taken a "stance pass" with both feet, start again, with the ball underneath the front of the foot. After positioning the ball underneath your foot, roll your foot over the ball (keeping the heel down), exposing the sides of the feet to the sensation of the ball. You can progress on a time frame that suits you best. The more you explore the soles of the feet with a rounded surface, the more you will gently stretch muscles and move joints in a way that is completely unique and novel, while completely natural!

Helpful Tips: If your feet are very stiff, start working your feet on the ball while sitting down. Sitting reduces how much weight is over the ball, which reduces the pressure. Once you notice improvement, you can increase the pressure by standing!

ATTENTION, OVERACHIEVERS!

The ball is a great place to start, so take a while learning and benefitting from this exercise. If you are highly motivated to increase the range of motion in the thirty-three joints of the foot, you can take it to the next level. A few companies have come out with stone walking mats. Just like they sound, these mats have smooth stones glued or sewn to them, allowing you to practice walking on a cobbled surface without necessarily needing to bare it all outside. If you find walking on the stones to be too big of a step from a tennis ball, try laying out a bath towel (or two) over the stones to build up the smaller muscles in the feet. This will decrease the intensity of the surface, allowing you to adapt to it more slowly.

Key Points, Chapter 8

1. Create a safe "barefoot" environment before beginning your foot health program.
2. Try each of the exercises to see how you do on your first pass. Which are easy and which are challenging?
3. Take your time on the exercises that are the most challenging, based on how they feel to your body.
4. Increasing the time spent on each exercise and the number of times each exercise is repeated, or changing the angles of your body to make the stretches more challenging are all ways of increasing the intensity of the program.

CHAPTER 9

Taking the Next (First) Step

"You have brains in your head.
"You have feet in your shoes.
"You can steer yourself in any direction you choose."
—Dr. Seuss

As we approach the end of this book, you may be facing a quandary. You understand all the information I've given. You no longer desire to have foot pain (did you *ever* desire to have foot pain?), but perhaps you feel trapped, as many people do, between the desire for wellness and what seems like some big changes in habit. You have, after all, been wearing shoes, and possibly wearing high-impact shoes, for some time now. Below are some of the usual comments I hear floating around the hall after I lecture on the subject of the high-heel hangover. Do any of them resonate with you?

- I can't afford to replace my entire footwear wardrobe, nor alter all of my clothes, to accommodate a new heel height.
- I love my heels and I feel [short; heavy; dumpy; less elegant; less professional] without them.
- I can't find the time to add an entire foot-training program into my day.
- It's so much easier to fix my problems with a shot or surgery.

And then there's the bit about walking. I know, you've been walking around your entire life in a particular way and now I am asking you to *change* how you go about getting from one place to the other? The nerve!

Believe it or not, I do not want you to feel overwhelmed. Feeling like there is a huge hurdle between you and health is only going to deter you from making the small (really!) changes that will give you relief. As a culture that likes to go big, we tend to attempt huge changes to our habits when we want to get better. When we want to lose weight, we go on ten-day fasts and eliminate all foods that start with "carb" from our diet. When we decide to start exercising, we go out and buy a three-year membership to a gym, a new pair of $200 running shoes, and five great workout outfits. What's the problem in these scenarios?

The change is too much and we are setting ourselves up to fail.

When we aren't eating well, the best solution for long-term success is to start by dropping one thing, like soda. Or the fourth cup of coffee. Ready to start exercising? Try a daily mile-long walk and take it from there. Stressed? The solution is not, realistically, moving to India for a forty-day retreat at your favorite ashram, but rather sitting still, with no cell phones, no talking, and no fidgeting for, let's say, ten minutes. Try it.

It is this overzealous approach to health that causes us to crash and burn like a kid after his Halloween candy binge. So I'm asking you to look at starting foot care in an easy-to-do way. Actually, you have already made improvements to your health by simply reading this book. One of the biggest cycles we get ourselves into with chronic pain is feeling like we are a victim to it. Suddenly, we become aware that most chronic conditions of the foot are a result of our own choices, and the lightbulb comes on. It's a great start.

Then, when you're ready, try out a few of the exercises. I don't recommend you start by doing them for thirty to forty minutes a day. This isn't a fitness manual, but a guide to testing out the muscles in your feet. It's alignment, and it doesn't require large amounts of physical effort. Each of the exercises can be done in one-minute increments throughout the day. I understand that finding a large gap in your schedule is challenging, so try running through a few of the exercises while brushing your teeth in the morning and evening.

Many of the guidelines given in this book can apply to things you are already doing. Paying attention to your gait pattern while out for your regular walk does not take any extra time, only a little extra attention. The same goes for adjusting your alignment while standing around in line at the bank or the grocery store. You can improve the health of your feet in seconds, simply by adjusting how you load them.

HOW OFTEN, AND FOR HOW LONG, DO I NEED TO DO THE EXERCISES?

At some point in our recent cultural history we developed a differentiation between exercise and movement. Exercise, by definition, requires a structured set of time, a level of intensity, a quantity of reps per session, and a number of sessions per week. The problem with thinking of alignment as a series of "exercise sessions" is that it implies that you don't have to think about where your body is in space all of the time, or at least, as often as possible. In order to change something as ingrained as how you use your body, you have to think while you are using your body. And that means you have to think about your alignment often, going beyond the time you are doing the exercises.

Now that I have said that, there are general guidelines that will help you change your tissue sooner, rather than later:

- You should work up to holding each exercise for at least a minute. This might not be possible at first. You may find that your muscles cramp and protest, which is a fairly normal part of any exercise program. Use your body's reactions to the exercise as a guide for increasing or decreasing the intensity or the duration of each hold.

- The more frequently you do the exercise, the better results you will have. The minimum for each exercise should be at least once a day, but a good middle-of-the-road habit to get into is cycling through the entire series of movements three times. Each time you run through the cycle, you will find the improvements to one set of muscles make it easier the second and then third time. Use the exercise section at the end of this book for easy reference.

- Learn the gait alterations and the basics of each stretch, and integrate them into your lifestyle, permanently. You will more than likely be a shoe-wearer for the rest of your life, which means you will need to keep some sort of exercise program going for your feet for, well, forever! Keep in mind that the muscles in your feet are made of the same exact tissue as the muscles in the rest of the body. You don't think the weight lifting you did ten years ago is still doing your body good, do you? The same muscle science applies to the feet, so keep up the good work!

WHEN WILL I FEEL BETTER?

The answer to this question is…it depends. The time it takes for your muscles to strengthen or restore in length depends on:

- What shape your feet are in now.

- The type of shoes you have worn throughout your life.
- The length of time you have been wearing shoes.
- Your particular gait pattern.
- How frequently you do your exercises.
- How frequently you think about and respond to where you carry your weight on your feet.
- The types of shoes, or the lack thereof, you choose moving forward.

For many ailments, the pain relief is immediate. If you have had the habit of bearing all of your weight on a particular area of your foot, to the point that you have developed an issue, just removing that weight will reduce pressure and change the situation in an instant.

Other ailments were created over years, or even decades. You can change your mechanics and make improvements on a cellular level that may not become apparent for years, although you likely will experience a gradual lessening of pain in the meantime. Whatever your experience is, know that whatever your original goal may have been (curing a chronic foot condition, for example), a new goal can be investing a small amount of time every day into ensuring healthier feet for the future.

When you start any exercise program, it is important to have small progress markers along the way. If you set a twenty-pound weight loss as a goal, and lose only twelve pounds, would that make your program ineffective? Of course not. Apply that same mentality to the goals you set with your feet.

When coping with pain, it is common to see changes in frequency, intensity, and even location.

FREQUENCY: How often are you experiencing pain?

INTENSITY: On a scale of one to ten, is your pain changing, or is it staying exactly the same?

LOCATION: Is your pain in the same area, or does that area feel better but now you are feeling pain in new areas of your foot or lower leg?

Use these as markers to measure if your new program or footwear is having an impact on your foot status.

MAKING OVER YOUR CLOSET

Whether you are considering changing 10 percent of your habits, or if you are excited enough to be thinking about changing out your entire closet, I have done my job well.

After reading through the suggestions and recommendations, you will find that it is not a requirement to toss out all of your footwear in order to get pain relief.

If you are ready to purchase footwear matching the guidelines appropriate to your feet (see Chapter 5), I suggest getting a pair in which you will do the greatest amount of walking. Your habits of walking are where you'll find your most ingrained movement patterns. You may be tempted to splurge on a pair of super-cute, flat dress shoes that will be worn once or twice a week while sitting at your desk, instead of getting the flexible, negative-heeled walking shoes to use on your thrice-weekly two-mile walk. Choose the latter. Whatever shoe you will wear the most often while bearing the brunt of your weight is the best choice for your dollar. If you can get both, then get both. If you can get neither, then take a good look at your closet, find the lowest, most acceptable heel to you right now, with the widest toe box, of course, and make that shoe your staple. And, do your exercises every day.

> *I got my first pair of high heels at age thirteen and I thought I was just too cute, until an older guy laughed at me for being so wobbly. Devastated but determined, I practiced wearing them and finally succeeded—I even was able to run in them. I couldn't figure out why I kept getting backaches and finally a herniated L5-S1 disc (duh). Went to chiropractic college to learn about the spine and learned about those wicked, but seductive, high heels. Bye-bye heels, although I, too, have a few pairs I hide in the closet that call to me in the night.*
>
> —GAYLE I., Chiropractor

I am often asked, "Do you ever wear heels? Ever?" I will admit that I keep a pair of gold, strappy heeled sandals in my closet. I bought them more than ten years ago and every time I spring clean, rearrange my closet, or move, I consider tossing them out. But I never do. These shoes make me feel like a Greek goddess when I imagine myself wearing them. I pick the outfit out in my mind, including the dress, jewelry, and the hair. In my Greek fantasy, my hair is down to the floor in perfect ringlets, just in case you were wondering.

All of this is true, actually. And so is this: I haven't actually worn these heels in five years. The first reason is, nowhere in my fantasy do the soles of my feet burn at the halfway point of the evening, or do I have to take off the shoes and put on a pair of scuffed backup shoes I found in the trunk of my car. Yet, both of these things usually happen whenever I wear heels.

I also happen to see a lot (and I mean a lot) of people who can no longer walk without pain due to the state of their feet. This inability to walk has translated into weight gain, or extended periods of time where the Unfortunate Sole (get it?) has battled depression due to the constant pain with every step.

I have worked with seniors who are unable to maintain functional lives due to the fact that their stiff and painful feet have jeopardized their balance, to the point of being at risk for a fall simply by walking through their house. Many people I have seen consider hip and knee replacements, foot surgery, and cortisone injections as the norm.

Frankly, I want more than that out of my physical experience. I would rather enjoy walking along the beach, using the power generated by my own muscles, for as long as possible. I want long-term function more than I want to live out my fashion fantasy that comes with the price of joint replacements, chronic pain, and impaired mobility. The good thing is we all have that choice!

My personal footwear choices are being barefoot often, using the "barefoot shoes" for walking and hiking as often as I can, and wearing negative heels or flats the rest of the time. I also spend a lot of time walking in alignment and doing my alignment exercises on a daily basis.

You will develop the program length and footwear closet that suit you best, using the way you feel as a marker for how diligent you have, or need, to become. Health is just like an outfit; you can style it however you'd like, so long as it makes you feel good!

ALIGNMENT, THE BIGGER PICTURE

You have learned about your feet and the importance of keeping them aligned for the sake of optimal physiological function and minimal degeneration. Even though this concept is applied to the topic of foot pain, the theory applies equally across the entire body.

There are so many ailments that stem from the limitations that we have placed on our bodies, either structurally (as those provided by shoes), or from our habits. These habits include either a lack of total-body movement, or an over-dependence on limited muscular patterns.

To some people, alignment solutions seem too simple to actually work. The reality is that fixing your alignment addresses your foot ailments at the root of the problem, and that's why converts are seeing real, positive changes in their bodies, despite years of seeking expensive treatments.

Don't get me wrong. I believe there is an appropriate place for expensive and complex treatments, but these should fall in line after eliminating the most basic, mechanical causes of everyday, so-called "ailments of affluence." The information in this book is basic—a sort of Practical Human Body 101. This was just about your feet. Imagine what the full volume set would teach you!

Key Points, Chapter 9

1. You absolutely do not need to scrap all the shoes in your closet to improve your current state of foot health.

2. If you need to purchase a shoe that is aligned with healthy-shoe criteria (see Chapter 5), pick a model that you will be wearing while logging most of your weekly walking miles.

3. Your rate of improvement is a function of how much time you spend breaking old habits and starting new, better habits of body use.

4. Your alignment matters to the health of you entire body, way more than most people understand.

5. Changing mechanical causes of ailments is a fairly simple, easy, and inexpensive way to begin searching for your relief.

CHAPTER 10

Guidelines, Recommendations, and Frequently Asked Questions

The following pages are an of integration of everything this book has covered, and how to use the information to make logical, healthy decisions when it comes to footwear and foot care. So let's start from the beginning—the very beginning...

A good timeline for foot health and development should begin at childhood, one would think. However, because so much of a child's development hinges on what the parent is doing, I like to start my recommendations at pregnancy because it is never too early to start modeling good behavior. Also, reading through this timeline may help you figure out (if you haven't already) where your personal foot experience was affected along the way.

A BABY ON THE WAY

Let's talk for a moment about pregnancy. Let's talk about the extra weight, all loaded on the midsection. The lack of flexibility, the difficulty putting on shoes, and the swollen ankles. I might also mention the back pain and pregnancy-induced sciatica, so very common these days. And I won't mention the nausea, so fresh in my mind (I'm writing this as I emerge from my first trimester).

All of these ailments, now a common part of pregnancy, actually are not a direct result of pregnancy, but a combination of extra weight loaded on a frame with altered geometry. With geometrical changes happening left and right, front and back, this is the perfect time to develop habits that don't make any musculoskeletal issue worse.

We now know that footwear affects joint position from the ankles all the way up to (and through) the spine. Putting these malaligned body parts under a steadily increasing weight will only make ailments of the foot (and lower leg) develop more quickly.

Other considerations specific to pregnancy are the potential changes to pelvic alignment that your footwear produce. When the pelvis is taken out of its natural alignment, the mobility of the muscles in the hips and pelvic girdle is affected, changing the mechanics of vaginal delivery. Creating unnatural changes in this area can lead to resistance in these muscles, which works against a natural, vaginal delivery.

For the sake of comfort, health, and better mechanics before and during delivery, stick to negative or flat heels, and spend lots of time opening the muscles in the feet, lower leg, and back of the thigh. Also, an extra bonus to keeping your pelvis stacked over your hips (as opposed to wearing it out in front of you) during pregnancy is enjoying the extra support your skeleton can lend to the increasing mass, as opposed to letting the soft tissue of the body carry the load.

KIDS

Childhood is a great time to start integrating all of the information in this book. The problem is that you probably won't get around to reading this book until you have kids of your own. Or, maybe your children already have children of their own. Well, you can still offer lots of advice from this section to others on what they should be doing with their kids. People love that, right?

Before picking out the perfect footwear for your children, it is important that I clearly state, there is no footwear required for correct foot development. Those of you who grew up in households where footwear was mandatory—"make sure you have your shoes on before you go outside!"—will be surprised. Yes, the human foot develops quite nicely, and likely even better, without shoes. This is despite my own painful memory of having a fish hook taken out of my foot in the middle of a camping trip, and a less painful memory (for me) of my sister stepping onto a nail sticking out of a board (she was about ten years old, on the phone with a boy, and no, she didn't even drop the phone). The reality is, the barefoot time required for natural foot development isn't always the safest option when we're surrounded with man-made surfaces and detritus.

The best solution I have found is to look for special children's brands that offer extreme flexibility, as well as lots of space to spread their toes. Keep in mind that children grow extremely fast, meaning that a shoe that fits today is swiftly on its way to becoming too small tomorrow. This gets expensive for sure. Many adults recollect squishing into hand-me-downs, or having to curl toes to prevent them from banging into their shoes by the end of the school year, and going barefoot in the summer before next year's shoes came in the fall. Buying shoes for the kids still tends to be dictated by the season rather than by the needs of the foot. The foot needs space!

When it comes to babies, they should not be put into shoes at all, especially when learning to walk. Since infants aren't walking around, foot coverings are usually needed for temperature control, which is fine. Pay attention, though. As infants begin to play with learning how to walk, a sock against a tile or hardwood floor inhibits development of the essential "push-off" part of human gait. Slick surfaces will cause a baby to develop an alternative to a natural gait pattern. Incorrect muscle pattern sequencing developed at an early age will stay with a person for life. Try to find socks or surfaces that offer traction, even if you have to create some nonslip socks in your sewing room. It is definitely worth it in the long run of natural movement development.

And, speaking of kids, it is frightening to see positive-heeled shoes on small children. Here's why: the body establishes the level of maximum bone mineral density by age twenty. The upright, weight-bearing motions that develop bone happen abundantly in kids—they've got a lot of energy and natural tendency to stay active. Putting a heel under their feet during this critical phase of bone development penalizes them for the rest of their life. You can never develop bone past the quantities set during this development phase. Do your kids a favor—forsake the trendy mini-fashions for their long-term skeletal longevity.

SHOES AT THE OFFICE

I do a lot of magazine interviews and reporters are always asking me for tips "for the woman who *has* to wear high heels." I am always happy to offer tips, but come on, who exactly is making you wear the heels? Seriously, if you've got "wearing heels" listed on your job contract, please send it to the Occupational Safety and Health Administration. That requirement shouldn't be there.

That said, if you wear heels because it makes you feel more professional, then you are going to have to do the exercises in this book on a more regular basis. The exercises are designed to help you lengthen all of the tissue most commonly shortened by certain parts of footwear. Keep in mind that the time you spend in shoes with geometry-altering components is the time you spend shortening all your pieces back up again.

If you are wearing positive-heeled shoes all the time—meaning not only are your work and casual shoes elevated above a flat but your athletic shoes have at least an inch under the back—you will find it takes a lot longer to get out of a foot crisis.

Here are some tips to quicken the pace:

- Get a pair of flat or negative-heeled walking shoes to ensure that your fitness-walking time improves not only your fitness level but also your foot health.
- Keep a pair of flats in your desk at work. When you find yourself needing to walk for an errand in the office, or if your feet end up feeling particularly limited in that day's shoes, slip on your backups. I have found that a pair of neutral, all-leather flats are suitable for most every outfit.
- Take a few three-to-five minute breaks within the workday, to do your exercises. To keep a copy of the exercises in your desk, use the tear-out portion of the exercise manual to help guide you.
- Get a pair of toe-alignment socks to slip on when you get home from work. This will give you a lot more time in the "spread-out" toe position than if just running through the exercises now and then.

AND FOR THE MEN

I know this is a book for the ladies, but like I said in Chapter 1, the basics of shoe parts, the laws of physics, and the theorems in geometry are not gender-biased! When purchasing footwear, men should be looking at the same things—the flexibility of the sole, the space for the toes, the ease with which the shoe stays on the foot, and, of course, the height of the heel.

> *I often wonder how many men have "bad backs" and traipse off to work in their heeled shoes—I have a swanky pair of men's dress shoes with heels that I like to wear to weddings. Which is ironic—the swanky part—since my back hurts so much by the time the reception starts that I take my shoes off for the dance floor before any of the women do. This begs the question, are men more wimpy than women, or just smarter when it comes to shoes?*
>
> —MICHAEL C.

The exercises, just like the footwear guidelines, are perfectly valid for men as well, so feel free to dig in!

SENIORS

Footwear research has tended to focus often on older adults. The reason? Foot pain has been shown to be associated with lack of mobility, balance, and self-efficacy in this population, and researchers want to know what can be done to improve the situation. One of the interesting findings in these studies is the prevalence of poor footwear fit, in both men and women. As tissues deform under years of loading (and misloading), the feet change in shape and size. The problem? Many seniors tend to wear the same shoes, or purchase new shoes without having their feet measured to see how their feet have changed.

It is often recommended that seniors begin purchasing shoes that offer large amounts of stability, meaning limited flexibility in the sole—very flat, very sturdy, etc. This suggestion is suitable for the senior who is not actively seeking to improve the health of her muscular system with regular exercise, balance therapy, or specific-movement classes. There is a fine line between creating a stable environment to avoid injury and impeding muscle development with the same measure.

A happy medium, I think, is to create a safe space for exercising barefoot and doing balance-improving exercise while using two main types of shoe. One should be less rigid for mindful sessions of gait improvement, and the other pair sturdier for times when multiple tasks make it difficult to pay attention to road surfaces, etc.

BONUS: A SIMPLE EXERCISE TO IMPROVE BALANCE

Stand in unshod feet, holding lightly to the back of a chair for support. Align the hips so they stack directly above the ankles. Make sure you can lift and wiggle the toes, demonstrating that your weight is far enough back over your heels.

Keeping both legs straight (it's very important that you don't bend either knee), push the right leg down into the floor, and let your left hip lift up away from the floor. Again (because I know how your knees want to cheat!), avoid bending the knees.

Keep your arms and shoulders relaxed and pay attention to how still (or not) your foot and ankle are. Practice this on a regular basis until you notice you are able to balance better and stay calm (relaxed shoulders, neck, face, etc.) while standing on one leg.

This is a simple exercise, but frankly, no one actually realizes how her stiff feet are contributing to her instability until she tests her balance!

ALL NATURAL, ALL THE TIME

What I like to call the "barefoot movement" has really taken off in the last few years due to some good books and magazine articles, and lots and lots of foot pain. People want to know *why* they are hurting, and it's about time someone started mentioning the fact that shoes have really done a number on the mechanics of the foot.

I really love the barefoot movement, but what I would have really, *really* loved would have been the barefoot movement starting about a hundred years ago, before it seemed like a good idea to lay down concrete and asphalt everywhere. The fact that our foot was not designed to wear shoes is self-evident. Another self-evident tidbit is that we humans require natural surfaces in order for our feet to handle walking without exceeding the natural limitations of soft and bony tissues.

We Westerners have a habit of picking a "natural" habit and jamming it into our unnatural lives, such as barefoot running for long distances on cement and asphalt. This takes a good thing (natural foot movement) and creates a vibrational loading that can lead to fractures in overloaded foot bones and injuries of the soft tissue. Train smart. Be logical. If you want natural foot movements for optimal health, walk in natural environments. Shoes have been protecting us from our overrigid environment for some time, and it takes time (years, even) to restore function. To get those feet healthier quicker, I strongly suggest a plan for increasing range of motion and function of the intrinsic foot musculature, and restoring appropriate length to extrinsic foot, lower leg, and thigh muscles.

I regularly see people get excited over the latest training fad, and run out and buy the new barefoot-simulating shoes so they can run in a way that is "better for their health." I see these same people take feet that have no motor skill or strength, slap on their new shoes, and take a long run on paved streets in their neighborhood, their upper body falling out in front of them, increasing the g-forces of their landing with every step. Slap! Slap! Slap!

You want to go *au naturel*? Here are some guidelines if you want to slowly transition yourself from a shoe-wearer to a minimalist.

1. Start with a daily stretching and massage of the heels, midfoot, forefoot, and toes.

2. Do your foot exercises—a lot. No, really, I mean it. Do them *all the time.*

3. Understand that the position of the foot is maintained by the muscles of the hips and make sure you optimize lateral hip (iliotibial or "IT" band), hamstring, gluteal, and adductor (inner thigh) strength with stretching and full ranges of motion. Tight hips limit foot function.

4. Get a superflexible shoe with minimal (or better yet, no) heel.

5. Before jumping into nonshoe shoes, deal with your whole-body alignment and gait mechanics. Podiatrists are seeing a huge increase in forefoot fractures from people (even highly experienced runners) who land with excessive force on the front of the foot. Walking should be heel to toe, not landing on the front of the foot. Running should be done on natural surfaces with body weight stacked correctly (without the torso leaning forward).

6. If you get nonshoe shoes, be a walker. If you do choose to run, build up your walking mileage for at least a year before even considering running in them.

7. Log your miles on a natural surface, with elevation changes and rocky obstacles. The urban

jungle is not a natural walking surface, and the friction and traction of this surface coupled with the lack of its yield can be quite damaging to the human body.

An interesting note: Barefoot parks, or outdoor areas that are dedicated for offering debris-free trails, pebbly surfaces, and plenty of in-nature, balance-challenging obstacles are beginning to pop up as more people become aware of our waning foot strength. Currently these parks are available mostly in Europe, but hopefully in time their importance will be recognized and developed in schools and public parks throughout the entire shoe-wearing world.

FAQs

As we come to the end of the book, there are a few questions that I tend to always get regarding feet, footwear, and special considerations. Hopefully your question is found somewhere on these pages!

Is There Ever a Right Time For...?

Flip-Flops

Sure. As basic foot protection in a public bathing area, getting in and out of the pool, or walking down on the beach, these bikini-esque shoes are great. The negative impact of this type of footwear only comes from wearing it often, creating certain muscular recruitment.

If you like the open feel of a flip-flop, try to find a shoe with a minimal, yet well-engineered upper that gives you plenty of breathing room across the feet without invoking alterations in your stride or your foot-firing patterns. There are many outdoor-shoe companies that strive to offer in-and-out-of-the-water footwear that makes water sports and outdoor activities safe for the feet, yet a lot more comfortable than a full, heavy shoe.

High Heels

I am sure by this point you think I hate fashion. Well, that's not true at all. I love cute shoes just as much as the next person. I just happen to love geometry a whole lot more. High-heeled shoes are fine to wear on those special occasions. Again, it is just the enduring habit of wearing these shoes that racks up the long-term damage. If you do happen to take the shoes out for a night on the town, you are more than likely going to have a High Heel Hangover to deal with the next day.

For feet not used to wearing killers, the hangover can be blisters, burning in the front of the foot, sore toes, tender lower legs, calf cramps, or next-day back pain. Give yourself time to do a few gentle passes over the exercises. To really loosen everything up, give yourself five minutes of foot exercise for every hour you spent in your shoes. When done, the skin of the feet may still be sensitive, but the muscles should feel a whole lot better.

P.S. If you happen to sprain your ankle while wearing these shoes, it is best not to tell me. I'll only say "I told you so," and then tell you to do your exercises once it heals.

What about Orthotics?

When foot tissues fail to maintain their structural integrity, that can allow structures to displace—the ankles, for example. Because the ankles are at the bottom of a long chain of other joints, moving them out of alignment can create a chain reaction that impacts the knees and hips.

Moving the hips out of alignment affects the musculature of the pelvic floor, the abdominals, and the spine, as many of these muscles attach to the bones in the legs.

As you can tell from this book, if the feet aren't doing their job, it is really important to rectify the situation. Orthotics are one way to prevent the entire structure from collapsing. However, the orthotic is not a foot-strengthening apparatus. The orthotic is essentially a support for the bones in lieu of the muscles doing their job.

Because you've read this deeply into the book, you will probably realize that I am about to tell you that in addition to using your orthotics, you will also need to undertake a foot-strengthening program.

I've Been Wearing Heels for a Long Time. Is It Safe to Drop Down into Flats?

Truthfully, if you have been wearing a high, positive-heeled shoe for a long time, it will take some time before your tissue releases enough to allow you to wear lower shoes comfortably and safely. Long before changing footwear, you can start the foot exercise program, gradually preparing your tissue. Stretching the calves is a real eye-opener for most people. If you can barely stretch your calves using the stretch from this book, you can wait a while before changing shoes.

That said, find the lowest heel height you feel comfortable in and set that as your new "highest" heel. You can start working your way down from that height, making progress that is accordant to the time you spend retraining your foot muscles and paying attention to your gait pattern.

Why Is My Doctor Prescribing Heels for my Plantar Fasciitis?

This is an old solution to the problem of extreme tension in the lower leg, Achilles tendon, and sole of the foot. The rationale is your tissues are so tight that simply dropping your heel down to the floor during the regular gait cycle is enough to tear the tissue. The short-term solution is to wear shoes that prevent your heel from getting to the ground. Being a short-term solution, it doesn't actually fix the problem, it just gets rid of the pain.

Continuing with a tension-making gait pattern that incorrectly loads foot and lower-leg tissues, the problem continues to worsen until you are right back where you started—suffering the pain of plantar fasciitis.

What to do? If you are currently unable to walk without a heel, see the recommendation above for those who have been wearing heels for a long time. The secret to dealing successfully with this issue is diligence—both in doing the exercises regularly, and in paying attention to how you carry your body over your feet while walking and standing.

What if I Want to Wear Shoes That Are Good for My Feet Most of the Time, but Still Keep Some of My Old Habits? Will That Make any Difference at All?

Keep in mind that the changes brought about by the high heel are similar to the physiological changes brought about by a really delicious dessert, like crème brûlée. Just because you eat crème brûlée every now and then doesn't mean that you've abandoned eating well most of the time. The same goes for footwear. When you splurge, it is just that—a splurge. Come home and work it off in the foot gym. A pair of flat or negative-heeled shoes are doing good whenever they are on your feet and nothing can take that away from you, not even a stroll down the shoe-candy aisle every now and then!

Key Points, Chapter 10

1. Footwear should always be selected thoughtfully, but there are certain stages of development where shoes can impact structures beyond the feet.

2. Selecting appropriate footwear for children is important, as this is the time when they are developing habits and tissues that will last them a lifetime.

3. There is a right time and right place for all footwear, but there is also a corresponding need to deal with aftereffects using exercise and other suggestions.

4. Because each of us has a unique "user's pattern" in our feet, the exercise program should be modified based on where you are right now, with a change in footwear happening gradually—especially in those with deeply ingrained foot-tension patterns.

EXERCISE AND POSITIONS TO KEEP HEALTHY FEET

FEET STRAIGHT

- Line up the OUTSIDE EDGE of each foot with a straight edge, like a plank in a wood floor.
- If this points your toes toward your midline, don't worry; they will adjust to their correct position with time and practice.

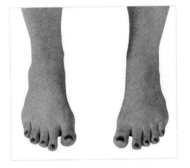

ANKLE TO HIP ON A
VERTICAL LINE

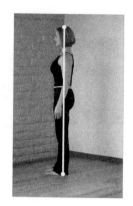

- Standing sideways to a mirror, hold a yardstick perpendicular to the ground (showing a vertical line).
- Still sideways, position your ankle to the bottom of the stick, and bring the center of your pelvis onto the line.
- Keep your knees straight, but kneecaps down.

MOVE THE TOES
INDIVIDUALLY

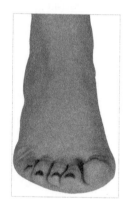

- Start by raising the big toe without moving any of the other toes.
- Then raise the second, third, fourth, and fifth, one at a time.
- Like you can move your fingers, practice moving your toes individually (or practice trying!).

STRETCHING THE CALVES

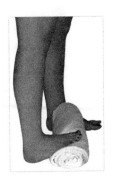

- Feet pointed straight ahead.
- Heel on the ground.
- Hips stay vertical over back ankle.

STRETCH YOUR TOES

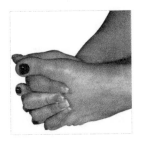

- Grab your left foot with your right hand, and vice versa.
- For more stretch, lace your fingers deeper between the toes, closer to the foot.

FOOT ON BALL

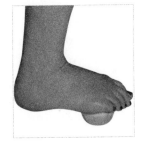

- Stand (or sit for less pressure) with your feet side by side.
- Keep your heel on the ground and press your forefoot onto a tennis ball. For a greater stretch, use a golf ball.
- Move the ball to different parts of the sole, applying continuous pressure. Hold each location for twenty to thirty seconds.

FORWARD FOLD
AGAINST A WALL

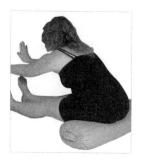

- Sit on a rolled towel or cushion, keeping the knees and thighs relaxed and straight.
- Press your heels into the wall.
- Reach your hands to the wall, folding at the level of the hips instead of along the spine.
- Take relaxing breaths, and do not bounce.

LENGTHEN THE BACKS
OF THE LEGS

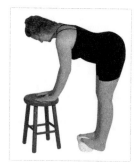

- Stand facing a chair with legs straight at the knees.
- Keep the feet straight, heels on the ground, forefeet raised onto a towel.
- Fold forward from the hips (not the spine) and let the tip of your tailbone rise up and away from the ground.

STRETCHING THE GRIPPING MUSCLES

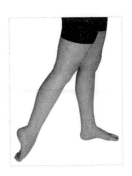

- Starting with the toenails, lay down the top of the foot behind you, keeping the heel centered.
- For more stretch, straighten the back knee and reach back from the hip.

SPREAD YOUR TOES

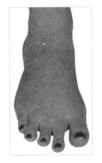

- Stand or sit with your feet pointed straight ahead.
- Practice spreading your toes away from each other—side to side, but not up or down.

APPENDIX

Many types of footwear and aids that might help you on your quest to improve your foot health were discussed in this book. For additional information on these products, please visit their websites listed below.

Footwear Brands

KALSO EARTH SHOES (NEGATIVE-HEELED SHOES)
www.earthbrands.com

SOCKWA
www.sockwa.com

SOFT STAR SHOES (GREAT CHILDREN'S LINE)
www.softstarshoes.com

VIBRAM ("BAREFOOT" SHOES)
www.vibramfivefingers.com/index.htm

Toe Alignment Socks

My-Happy Feet Original Alignment Sock
www.my-happyfeet.com

Cobblestone Walking Mats

Can be found at:
www.allegromedical.com
www.amazon.com
www.gaiam.com

Barefoot Walking Parks

www.barfusspark.info (Note: Select ENGLISH to translate page)

GLOSSARY OF TERMS

A

abduction: in anatomy, the movement of a limb or bone away from the midline of the body; abduction of both legs spreads the legs. The opposite of abduction is adduction.

abductor: a muscle or muscle group that moves a limb or bone away from the midline of the body

adduction: in anatomy, the movement of a limb or bone toward the midline of the body; adduction of the legs brings them together. The opposite of adduction is abduction.

ailments of affluence: diseases that are believed to be a result of increasing wealth or abundance within a society

alignment: the optimal position of an object (bones, in this case) to others (bone and joints) that maximizes function

arch of the foot: the shape of the foot's long axis that should be created by correct muscle contraction, bone orientation, and connective tissue lengths

atrophy: a wasting away of a tissue; in muscle, atrophy decreases the mass and leads to muscle weakness

B

ballistic: a type of stretching that includes "bouncing" on muscles that have not relaxed

biological sciences: a collection of information that deals with the study of life and living organisms

biomechanics: the study of the mechanical laws (see *Newtonian physics*) relating to the movement or structure of living organisms

biomechanist: one who studies the field of biomechanics

bone spur: an abnormal growth that creates a bony projection (also called an osteophyte), usually formed in response to incorrect rubbing, pressure, or stress

C

calf muscles: the group of musculature found at the back of the lower leg, and affecting the joints of the knee and ankle

center of mass: the mean location of all the mass in a system; if you were a ball (which you aren't), your center of mass would be found dead center. In standing humans, the center of mass is found in the pelvis.

circulation: movement in a regular or cyclic pattern, as the movement of the blood through the heart and blood vessels

collagen: the fibrous protein constituent of bone, cartilage, tendon, and other connective tissues

common: of frequent or familiar occurrence in a population, without regard to causality, desirability, or preventability

compensatory mechanisms: an action taken by the body to continue physiological function despite an alteration in natural function

connective tissue: a structurally simple type of biological tissue that connects, supports, or surrounds other tissues, organs, etc.

contraction: when a muscle works to become temporarily shortened, or bring its ends together

D

degeneration: deterioration or decline of a tissue over time

densest: most compact, having the most matter per volume

F

fascial systems: the network of structurally important and complex non-elastic tissues (fascia) that support, connect or hold internal body parts

femoral neck: the part of the femur (thigh bone) that veers toward the hip joint at an angle, and is typically where the break occurs in a hip fracture

"fit shoes": footwear that, in addition to covering the feet, purport to deliver additional fitness benefits such as muscle development, increased calorie expenditure, etc.

foot arch: see *arch of the foot*

fracture: a break in bone resulting from a trauma, excessive loading over time, or normal use of a compromised bone

friction: a force the resists the sliding motion of one object relative to another, like the ball of the hip rubbing on the socket of the hip joint

G

gait: the way you walk; refers to the sum of all the coordinated movements that create your pattern of walking

genetic: dictated by one's DNA

geometry: mathematical laws of angles; used by engineers and architects to ensure that a structure is able to withstand certain forces placed against it

gravity: the force that attracts the human body toward the surface of the earth; this pull is always along a vertical line

H

hamstrings: the group of musculature found at the back (posterior) of the thighs, and affecting the knees, hip joints and pelvis *"healthy shoes"*: footwear that, in addition to covering the feet, purport to deliver additional health benefits such as better balance or enhanced posture

hips: these are the two ball-and-socket joints where the tops of the legs meet the pelvis

I

inflamed: characterized by inflammation, a complex natural process of the body to heal an injury, infection, or irritation, characterized by redness and "burning" sensation

innervate: to "turn on" the nerves in an area of the body, which in turn will enable muscle contraction, lymph removal, etc.

K

kinesiology: the science of human movement

L

ligaments: fibrous, non-elastic bands of tissue that connect bones to each other, and serve as a sort of "fail-safe" to prevent a joint opening in a way that would create injury

loaded: positioned in such a way as to bear body weight

lumbar: the lowest part of the spine, just above the pelvis

M

metatarsals: the bones between the ankle (tarsals) and the toes (phalanges)

mobility: when describing a joint, the range of movement; when describing a person, the ability/freedom to move around on a daily basis

musculoskeletal: relating to the muscles and bones

N

natural: produced by or occurring in nature

neuropathy: disease or damage to a nerve that results in the dysfunction of the peripheral nerves

nervous system: the system of nerves and nerve centers in the body, including the brain and spinal cord

Newtonian Physics: the set of physical laws describing the motion of bodies under the action of a system of forces

O

objective markers: externally observable points of reference that show if the skeleton is stacked in a sustainable way, based on the laws of physics

organic tissue: the "stuff" that living things are made of

osteogenic or *osteogenesis*: the generation of bone

osteoporosis: a reduction in bone mineral density, compromising structural integrity of a bone and increasing the risk of a fracture or break

P

pelvic floor: a group of muscles in the pelvis that create the strong-yet-supple base of the torso and support the bladder, bowels, and pelvic organs

pelvis: the bowl-shaped bony structure that is located at in the lowest part of the torso, and is stacked onto the tops of the femurs, or thigh bones

pelvis thruster: someone who stands or walks in a posture that places the pelvis not stacked over the ankle, but suspended over the front of the foot

phalanges: the name of the bones contained entirely within the fingers or the toes

physical sciences: those natural sciences outside of biology; e.g. physics, chemistry

physiological: relating to the complex human functions that maintain homeostasis, or internal balance, of the human being

plantar fasciitis: painful inflammation of the plantar fascia (connective tissue in the bottom of the foot)

positive-heeled shoe: any shoe that places the back of the foot higher than the front

posterior leg muscles: those muscles that run down the backs of the upper and lower leg bones; see *hamstrings and calf muscles*

pressure: the effect that occurs when a force (like weight) is applied

propulsion: the act of moving a body forward

R

regeneration: in biology, the process of replacing with new growth those tissues or cells that are impaired, damaged, or dead

S

sacroiliac joints: the points of connection between the sacrum and the pelvis, in the lower back

spinal cord: the thick bundle of nerves that runs through the spinal column and serves as the main highway of communication between the brain and the rest of the body

spinal column: a term used to describe the bones that form the spine

spinal disks (or discs): the anatomical, gel-filled pillow-like structure between the vertebrae (bones in the spine)

stabilized: in the musculoskeletal system, refers to holding body parts in their correct position

stack vertically: to position the bones of the body while standing so as to create minimal sway forward, backward, or sideways

symmetry: the use or positioning of both sides of the body equally

T

tailbone: informal name for the coccyx, or bones found at the very bottom of the spine

tendons: fibrous tissues that connect muscles to bones

thoracic spine: the middle part of the spine, from the last rib up to just below the neck

thighs: the common term for the muscles packed around the bone of the upper leg (femur)

tissue: a collection of cells in the body serving a common purpose; examples include muscular, skeletal, nerve, connective, etc.

torso: the trunk of the body; excludes arms, legs, and head

U

unshod: without shoes

V

vertical: at right angles (perpendicular) to a horizontal plane, in this case the surface of the earth; the vertical stacking of the body means that that the top is directly above the bottom.

W

weight-bearing: when a structure is carrying the full burden of its own mass; in the human case, when the bones are holding the vertical mass of the body

FOR FURTHER READING

THE BARE FOOT

Bergmann, G., H. Kniggendorf, F. Graichen, and A. Rohlmann. 1995. Influence of shoes and heel strike on the loading of the hip joint. *Journal of Biomechanics* 28 (7): 817-27.

Daoût, K., T. Pataky, D. De Clercq, and P. Aerts. 2009. The effects of habitual footwear use: foot shape and function in native barefoot walkers. *Footwear Science*: 1 (2): 81-94.

De Wit, B., D. De Clercq, and P. Aerts. 2000. Biomechanical analysis of the stance phase during barefoot and shod running. *Journal of Biomechanics* 33 (3): 269-78.

Nigg, B. 2001. The role of impact forces and foot pronation: a new paradigm. *Clinical Journal of Sports Medicine* 11 (1): 2-9.

Rao, U., and B. Joseph. 1992. The influence of footwear on the prevalence of flat foot. A survey of 2300 children. *The Journal of Bone and Joint Surgery* 74 (4): 525-27.

Robbins, S., and A. Hanna. 1987. Running-related injury prevention through barefoot adaptations. *Medicine and Science in Sports and Exercise* 19 (2): 148-56.

Robbins, S., G. Gouw, and A. Hanna. 1989. Running-related injury prevention through innate impact-moderating behavior. *Medicine and Science in Sports and Exercise* 21 (2): 130-39.

Rome, K., D. Hancock, and D. Poratt. 2008. Barefoot running and walking: the pros and cons based on current evidence. *The New Zealand Medical Journal* 121 (1272).

Rossi, W.A. 1999. Why Shoes Make 'Normal' Gait Impossible. *Podiatry Management* (March): 50-61.

Rossi, W.A. 2001. Footwear: the primary cause of foot disorders. Podiatry Management (February): 129-38.

von Tscharner, V., B. Goepfert, and B. Nigg. 2003. Changes in EMG signals for the muscle tibialis anterior while running barefoot or with shoes resolved by non-linearly scaled wavelets. *Journal of Biomechanics* 36 (8):1169-76.

Vormittag, K., R. Calonje, and W.W. Briner. 2009. Foot and ankle injuries in the barefoot sport. *Current Sports Medicine Reports* 8 (5): 262-66.

Willems, T., E. Witvrouw, A. De Cock, and D. De Clercq. 2007. Gait-related risk factors for exercise-related lower-leg pain during shod running. *Medicine and Science in Sports and Exercise* 39 (2): 330-39.

Zipfel, B. and L.R. Berger. 2007. Shod versus unshod: the emergence of forefoot pathology in modern humans. *The Foot* 17 (4): 205-13.

Howell, L.D. *The Barefoot Book: 50 Great Reasons to Kick Off Your Shoes* by L. Daniel Howell. ISBN: 9780897935548.

BUNIONS

Barnett, C. 1962. The normal orientation of the human hallux and the effect of footwear. *Journal of Anatomy* 96 (Part 4): 489–94.1.

Barnicot, N.A. 1955. The position of the hallux in West Africans. *Journal of Anatomy* 89 (Part 3): 355–61.

Cho, N.H., S. Kim, D.J. Kwon, and H.A. Kim. 2009. The prevalence of hallux valgus and its association with foot pain and function in a rural Korean community. *Journal of Bone and Joint Surgery*—British Volume 91 (4): 494-98.

Gottschalk F., J. Sallis, P. Beighton, and L. Solomon. 1980. A comparison of the prevalence of hallux valgus in three South African populations. *South African Medical Journal* 57 (10): 355-57.

Maclennan, R. 1966. Prevalence of hallux valgus in a neolithic New Guinea population. *The Lancet* 287 (7452): 1398-1400.

Nix, S., M. Smith, and B. Vicenzino. 2010. Prevalence of hallux valgus in the general population: a systematic review and meta-analysis. *Journal of Foot and Ankle Research* 3 (September 27): 21.

FLIP-FLOPS

Carl, T., and S. Barrett. 2008. Computerized analysis of plantar pressure variation in flip-flops, athletic shoes, and bare feet. *Journal of the American Podiatric Medical Association* 98 (5): 374-78.

Shroyer, J., and W. Weimar. 2010. Comparative analysis of human gait while wearing thong-style flip-flops versus sneakers. *Journal of the American Podiatric Medical Association* 100 (4): 251-57.

FOOTWEAR CHARACTERISTICS
AND FOOT PAIN, AILMENTS

Arnadottir, S., and V. Mercer. 2000. Effects of footwear on measurements of balance and gait in women between the ages of 65 and 93 years. *Physical Therapy* 80 (1): 17-27.

Dawson, J., M. Thorogood, S. Marks, E. Juszczak, C. Dodd, G. Lavis, and R. Fitzpatrick. 2002. The prevalence of foot problems in older women: a cause for concern. *Journal of Public Health* 24 (2): 77-84.

de Lateur, B., R. Giaconi, K. Questad, M. Ko, and J. Lehmann. 1991. Footwear and posture: compensatory strategies for heel height. *American Journal of Physical Medicine Rehabilitation* 70 (5): 246-54.

Frey, C., F. Thompson, J. Smith, M. Sanders, and H. Horstman. 1993. American Orthopaedic Foot and Ankle Society women's shoe survey. *Foot and Ankle* 14 (2): 78-81.

Fulkerson, J., E. Arendt, L. Griffin, J. Garrick. 2002. Anterior knee pain in females. *Clinical Orthopaedics & Related Research* 372 (March): 69-73.

Hill, C., T. Gill, H. Menz, and A. Taylor. 2008. Prevalence and correlates of foot pain in a population-based study: the North West Adelaide health study. *Journal of*

Foot and Ankle Research, July 28, 2008. http://www.ncbi. nlm.nih.gov/pmc/articles/PMC2547889/.

Menz, H.B., and M.E. Morris. 2005. Footwear characteristics and foot problems in older people. *Gerontology* 51 (5): 346-51.

Menz, H.B., A. Tiedemann, M.M. Kwan, K. Plumb, and S.R. Lord. 2007. Foot pain in community-dwelling older people: an evaluation of the Manchester Foot Pain and Disability Index. *Rheumatology* (Oxford) 46 (2): 375.

Rossi, W. 2001. Footwear: The primary cause of foot disorders. A continuation of the scientific review of the failings of modern shoes. *Podiatry Management* (February).

Sherrington, C., and H. Menz. 2002. An evaluation of footwear worn at the time of fall-related hip fracture. *Age and Aging* 32 (3): 310-14.

HIGH HEELS

Bendix, T., S. Sorensen, and K. Klausen. 1984. Lumbar curve, trunk muscles, and line of gravity with different heel heights. *Spine* 9 (2): 223-27.

Csapo, R., C. Maganaris, O. Seynnes, and M. Narici. 2010. On muscle, tendon and high heels. *Journal of Experimental Biology* 213:2582-88.

Eisenhardt, J., D. Cook, I. Pregler, and H. Foehl. 1996. Changes in temporal gait characteristics and pressure distribution for bare feet versus various heel heights. *Gait and Posture* 4 (4): 280-86.

Esenyel, M., K. Walsh, J. Walden, and A. Gitter. 2003. Kinetics of high-heeled gait. *Journal of the American Podiatric Medical Association* 93 (1): 27-32.

Gabell, A., M. Simons, and U. Nayak. 1985. Falls in the healthy elderly: predisposing causes. *Ergonomics* 28 (7): 965-75.

Gefen, A., M. Megido-Ravid, Y. Itzchak, and M. Arcan. 2001. Analysis of muscular fatigue and foot stability during high-heeled gait. *Gait and Posture* 15 (1): 56-63.

Kerrigan, D., J. Johansson, M. Bryant, J. Boxer, U. Croce, and P. Riley. 2005. Moderate-heeled shoes and knee joint torques relevant to the development and progression of knee osteoarthritis. *Physical Medicine and Rehabilitation* 86 (5): 871-75.

Kerrigan, D., J. Lelas, and M. Karvosky. 2001. Women's shoes and knee osteoarthritis. *The Lancet* 357 (9262): 1097-98.

Kerrigan, D., M. Todd, and P. Riley. 1998. Knee osteoarthritis and high-heeled shoes. *The Lancet* 351 (9113): 1399-1401.

Lee, C., E. Jeong, and A. Freivalds. 2001. Biomechanical effects of wearing high-heeled shoes. *International Journal of Industrial Ergonomics* 28 (6): 321-26.

McBride I., U. Wyss, T. Cooke, L. Murphy, J. Phillips, and S. Olney. 1991. First metatarsophalangeal joint reaction forces during high-heel gait. *Foot and Ankle.* 11 (5): 282-88.

ABOUT THE AUTHOR

Katy Bowman is the first scientist of human physics to direct her expertise to the modern health crisis. Katy is a master's level Biomechanist and has taught tens of thousands to identify and repair the causes of disease that are mechanical, as opposed to hormonal or genetic. She teaches from a unique platform—one that is truly holistic, unfailingly scientific and with the compassion necessary to truly open people's minds.

With her trademark humor and incisive mind, Katy teaches health professionals, as well as the general public, to deal with female pelvic floor disorder, bone regeneration, and foot diseases. Her astonishingly simple corrective programs provide the sort of relief generally considered to be impossible.

Katy is a full-time mother, and directs the on-line programming of the Restorative Exercise Institute. She is the producer and talent of the Aligned and Well DVD line, lectures around world, and blogs regularly. She is very tired - but always happy!

She and her family split their time between their farm (and new alignment center) on Washington state's Olympic Peninsula, and the "ground zero" of wellness-through-alignment, in Ventura, California.

IMAGE CREDITS

CHAPTER ONE:

All illustrations by Carol Gravelle.

CHAPTER TWO:

Page 28: Photo by Cecilia Ortiz. Model is Breena Maggio.
Page 29: Photos by Cecilia Ortiz. Model is Breena Maggio.
Pages 35–37: Photos from Katy Bowman's personal archive.

CHAPTER THREE:

Page 41: Photos by Brad Kazmerzak. Model is Katy Bowman.
Page 42: Photos by Brad Kazmerzak. Model is Katy Bowman.
Page 43: Photos by Brad Kazmerzak. Model is Katy Bowman.

All photos previously appeared in *LA Yoga Magazine*.

CHAPTER FIVE:

Page 57: Illustration by Carol Gravelle.

CHAPTER SIX:

Page 74: Illustration by Cecilia Ortiz, adapted from Rossi.
Page 79: Photo by Cecilia Ortiz. Model is Breena Maggio.

CHAPTER EIGHT:

Page 97: Photo by Cecila Ortiz. Model is Breena Maggio.

Page 98: Photos by Cecila Ortiz. Model is Breena Maggio.

Page 101: Photos by Cecila Ortiz. Model is Breena Maggio.

Page 102: Photo by Cecila Ortiz. Model is Breena Maggio.

Page 104: Photo by Cecila Ortiz. Model is Breena Maggio.

Page 105: Photo by Cecila Ortiz. Model is Breena Maggio.

Page 107: Photo by Cecila Ortiz. Model is Breena Maggio.

Page 108: Photos by Cecila Ortiz. Model is Breena Maggio.

Page 110: Photo by Cecila Ortiz. Model is Breena Maggio.

Page 111: Photo by Cecila Ortiz. Model is Breena Maggio.

Page 114: Photo by Cecila Ortiz. Model is Breena Maggio.

INDEX